Trekking Through Cancerland

Letters from the Journey

Karen Loss

The photo of the author and Michael Crawford on page 78 was provided by the Michael Crawford International Fan Association (MCIFA) and is used with their permission.

The female clown face graphic on page 53 is used under a merchandise license agreement with GL Stock Images, LLC.

WHAT READERS SAY ABOUT TREKKING

Please know you are in my thoughts and prayers and I am so proud of you for being so strong. You have a long road ahead, so if you have a moment or two of weakness, know that I am here for you and can help. – *GL-Virginia*

I am reassured by the way you are dealing with this. Your strength and sense of humor – rooted in your trust in Jesus is a testimony for all of us and an example of how to face this kind of trial. – *DD-California*

I know that you have been through many difficult times in your life, but the way that you handle it has been inspiring. Just like now, whether you know or not, your battle against cancer inspires me and others (I am certain) to live our lives with more thanks, more closeness to God, and more concern for others. – *AB-Virginia*

Your journals are incredible. They are a testament to your courage, your candor, your wisdom and intelligence, your grace, and your astounding equanimity. I feel privileged to read them and to be able to accompany you (through them) on this journey. – *AG-Virginia*

I think your timing is perfect on this. There are serious and to a degree somber thoughts and reflections that we would all go through, should we be in your shoes. You are right, we all have a purpose and gifts to give. – *CS-Florida*

You are so honest and I am so blessed and glad I have found friends who are willing to talk about the hard stuff. – *AR-Virginia*

I know it's not easy for you. I will be praying for you - to alleviate itches, and troublesome side effects, and that the treatment will be effective and you'll have years and years and years more to add your light to the lives of SOOO many. – *SR-Virginia*

Sounds like you are patiently accepting whatever comes and trusting God for your future. It is a great testimony to your faith, demonstrating that it is real and not just a sunny day affair. – *BO-Pennsylvania*

Thanks so much for sharing this part of your story! None of us are meant to be self-sufficient even in the best of times, much less while being systematically poisoned, albeit for a good cause. – *KH-Virginia*

Sometimes it takes greater bravery to face our fears and our sadness and our pain than to pull ourselves up by our bootstraps, shove the feelings aside, and buck up on the outside. – *BS-Illinois*

I always love to read your updates and feel encouraged by your continued positive outlook. That's half the battle. Your sense of humor is another of your weapons! – *DF-Pennsylvania*

I just listened to your song twice with a tear in my eye. It is so beautiful…you are a woman of many talents. Your positive attitude is so visible in your emails. Keep up the fight!!! – *CS-Massachusetts*

I have drunk in your "medical updates" and used them to guide me in boosting others in down moments. – *AG-Virginia*

Somehow, even in your darkest times, your humor and faith shine through and it is contagious! And while I am sure your goal in life has not been to be an inspiration to others, you are. – *BB-Virginia*

You've done a wonderful job of conveying all aspects of your journey in mind, body and spirit. It's a wonderful testament to your faith and to your fortitude. Not to mention entertaining! Now that's a rare gift to make cancer entertaining. – *MS-Virginia*

I, like you, don't really believe in coincidences. God's hand has been in this every step of the way- no matter how difficult. – *BB-Pennsylvania*

If I ever have to deal with something like this, I know the memory of how you've handled it will inspire me. Thank you for that! – *JE-Virginia*

In sharing your journey and medical updates you are offering a valuable insight to many aspects surrounding this disease. You are allowing God's Glory to shine through you. He never promised us we wouldn't have our trials but He did promise He would always be with us. – *CS-Florida*

God is using you to spread the unexplainable joy that can be experienced even in the darkest of situations. People who do not know of His incredible grace have to be looking at you and saying "I want what she has." – *B-J B-Virginia*

I think your faith in God has had the most influence over

your health. I'm not negating modern nor alternative medicine, however I believe faith is the key ingredient to any therapy. – *NC-Virginia*

Your thoughts give me comfort and perspective, when I think about my own mortality or even that of those close to me. – *JF-Pennsylvania*

Surely one of the reasons you're here is to teach others how to handle the really bad things in life with grace, patience, and humor. Reading your letters gives me the strength to go out there and write off the little things, and face the big ones! Thank you for that. – *LD-Virginia*

DEDICATION

I dedicate this book to my grandmother Carrie Grove and my mother Gerry Loss, two women who taught me to put my faith in God and how to persevere in the face of serious physical challenges.

CONTENTS

INTRODUCTION i

November 28, 2012 Diagnosis: That Fateful Phone Call... 1

December 4, 2012 Discussing Treatment Options 3

December 11, 2012 Negative EGFR Means Chemo
Coming 7

December 18, 2012 Chemo Class Prep 10

December 20, 2012 First Chemo Day Experience............ 14

December 30, 2012 Side Effects? 17

January 2, 2013 Going for My First Wig 21

January 10, 2013 Laryngitis, Neuropathy, and Itching, Oh
My 24

January 14, 2013 Bald and Beautiful 29

January 22, 2013 More on Side Effects 34

January 29, 2013 Impacts on Friends and Loved Ones.... 38

February 2, 2013 Halfway Through 42

February 7, 2013 Some Days ARE Hard 46

February 13, 2013 Taking a Makeup Class for Cancer
Patients 50

February 23, 2013 Mid-Term PET Scan Results 55

March 3, 2013 Michael Crawford and Doggy Snuggles ... 59

March 10, 2013 Itching to the Max and Hand Healing.... 63

March 18, 2013 Adding Herbal Treatments to My
Regimen 68

March 27, 2013 Meeting Michael 73

April 4, 2013 It is Finished (Chemo that is) 80

April 11, 2013 Awaiting PET Scan Results While Wearing New Hats.. 85

April 17, 2013 Hat Stories and Drippy Noses.................... 89

April 25, 2013 Praise God for Good Results 94

May 2, 2013 Yay…No Evidence of Metabolic Activity ... 97

May 8, 2013 The Object is to Maintain, Literally at a Cost 101

May 16, 2013 A Top Ten Finish 106

May 23, 2013 Connecting Dots and Wondering 111

June 2, 2013 BP Meds, Car Shopping and Open-Air Topping 115

June 10, 2013 Celebrating My New Car, Hatless and Scarfless 120

June 19, 2013 Another Avastin Appointment 124

June 29, 2013 Goodbye Tucker Tucson and Leveling with the Doc 128

July 13, 2013 Rocking Out with Sir Paul and Other Things 133

July 22, 2013 Celebrating My Birthday and Planning Trips 138

August 4, 2013 Odds and Ends... 142

August 8, 2013 Preparing My Mind and Soul 145

August 21, 2013 Good Results and Reflections on Life 149

EPILOGUE 153

INTRODUCTION

Lying there in bed, my mind drifted to an unexpected question. "How will I respond if ever I am diagnosed with cancer?" Why in the world would I think that? After all, I was in my early 30s. I felt fine. No immediate family member, and few extended family members, had dealt with any forms of cancer.

I wasn't fearful or anxious – just contemplative. And the funny thing was, this thought crept into my nighttime thoughts on a number of occasions over a few years between my early to mid 30s. During those occasional nights, I would deliberate. Having always been a bit of a stoic, I knew that I would want to stay strong, not so much for others but for myself. If I got bad news and went to pieces, it would only make me feel silly, however unwarranted that belief might be under such circumstances. And, if I stayed strong, what would come after the bad news had settled in?

Would I need surgery? Would I have to undergo chemotherapy? Radiation? Knowing my penchant for motion sickness, and the things I'd always heard about chemo, would unending days of nausea be a part of such a scenario for me? I didn't know, of course, but I thought about all of these things and more, some with a degree of trepidation.

How would my family react? And my friends? Could I share the Christian faith that sustains me with those around me? Would they understand? Might my life and response to cancer be a testimony to others of how to face life's challenges and come out ahead, even if it might still

i

mean walking toward the end of my earthly life? These were the questions I pondered in the nighttime nearly 20 years ago.

As it turned out, I wouldn't have too long to wait in the larger scheme of things. About midway through my 36th year, and just one year after I'd had a laparoscopy to deal with an ovarian cyst, I was notified that I likely had cancer. I had been treating since my outpatient cyst surgery with hormone pills, but about 8 months along, the treatment seemed to go haywire. I began bleeding profusely and contacted my doctor to determine the best course of action. She told me to stop the drugs, let my body reregulate itself, and we would take things from there.

This seemed to work fine initially. Over the next few months, however, I realized that while the bleeding had stopped, things were not proceeding according to the normal course for a woman of my age. When I had my annual checkup later that fall, the doctor told me things were not quite right, so she wanted me to schedule an ultrasound right away. She kept calm, but made it clear that I should not wait.

Within a week's time, I had the ultrasound. The technician, while not being allowed to offer diagnostic information to me, did let it be known, even if inadvertently, that she was seeing things that weren't normal. In fact, as it turned out, she could not see some of my internal organs at all because something was blocking them from view. By the time I returned to my office, I had already received a phone call from my doctor's office. I returned the call and learned that there was a good-sized tumor (13 ½ centimeters) inside of me, and they thought it was likely cancer.

This would knock anyone for a little loop, and I was a bit stunned with the news. I quickly went about setting up consultation appointments with gynecologic oncologists. Both the first and second doctor who examined me felt that the odds were about two to one that it was cancer, but that in any event, it had to come out. So, I chose the surgeon I would work with, scheduled surgery for January 7, 1997, and prepared for Christmas as I awaited this next phase of my life. For my reading "pleasure" during this time, I visited my local library and selected a book full of case studies written by other women who had faced reproductive system cancers. Wow! I soon realized that reading the material in that book was the best thing I could have done. It prepared me for every step in the journey ahead, and it took the fear and trepidation away.

Still not knowing the final diagnosis as I went into surgery early on that January morning, I was prepared to deal with whatever was to come. When I awoke hours later, I learned that the pathology reports were positive for cancer, but that it was early stage. In fact, there were two primary cancers…in the uterus and also in the ovaries. Neither had spread, and so to my pleasant and even grateful surprise, my surgeon opted not to send me into chemotherapy or radiation after surgery. I had many, many doctor visits in the next five years in order to keep a close eye on my progress. When I remained cancer-free throughout that period, I was finally declared healed.

In the ensuing years, I continued to be vigilant about having annual checkups and routine radiographic tests. My life was, in many respects, pretty run-of-the-mill. I worked, I traveled, I played, I exercised, I ate whatever I wanted. Nothing was off limits, and in most ways, I was chugging along just fine. Well, fine, that is, until perhaps sometime in 2009 when I began having what I have taken to calling "chest attacks." To this day, no one knows if those chest attacks were caused by the lung cancer that would not be diagnosed for another couple of years, but they did indeed bring about the eventual tests that found the cancer in November of 2012.

That diagnosis is where the letters in this book begin. Once I began telling friends and family of my diagnosis, interest grew. People wanted to know the details, and they wanted to know how they could help. Almost immediately, more than 100 people populated the emailing list, and over ensuing months, that grew to 150, then to 200, and well beyond. It heartens my soul to know that so many friends and relatives care and want to learn about the heartaches, challenges, triumphs, and even humor associated with Trekking Through Cancerland.

So, I invite readers to learn what my journey has been like as I have fought the battle against lung cancer, sometimes through raging skirmishes, sometimes across comical terrain, and other times by traveling over a lake of love produced by those surrounding and supporting me. I hope it may prove helpful to others who must face similar villains or those who care about someone who is facing them.

Karen Loss
January 2014

1

November 28, 2012
Diagnosis: That Fateful Phone Call

Hi folks,

Most of you know that I had a CT guided lung biopsy done last Wednesday to determine the cause of a spot that had showed up on my lower right lung in a recent CT scan. [According to MedicineNet.com: *Computerized (or computed) tomography, and often formerly referred to as computerized axial tomography (CAT) scan, is an X-ray procedure that combines many X-ray images with the aid of a computer to generate cross-sectional views and, if needed, three-dimensional images of the internal organs and structures of the body....A CT scan is used to define normal and abnormal structures in the body and/or assist in procedures by helping to accurately guide the placement of instruments or treatments.*] In that scan, another larger spot also showed up on my liver. About ½ hour ago I received the results of this biopsy and, unfortunately, it indicates a primary cancer in my lung. My doctor who sent me for these tests thinks the liver spot is likely related to it, as well as an "elevated" diaphragm which also showed up in the pictures. I've been able to schedule a consultation with a local oncologist recommended by my gastroenterologist for tomorrow morning at 8 a.m. to see what needs to be done in the days/weeks/months to come.

While I obviously knew this was a possibility, 40% chance in fact, in one of the online sources I checked, I must say that I did not really expect this result. Well, since I will now join the ranks of repeat cancer victims, all I can do is take this a day at a time and hope for the best. Feel free to tell anyone who knows me and who you believe should know. It will be no secret with me and I am willing to talk about it, so don't wonder about that. I'll keep you posted as I learn more, but would, of course, ask you to lift me up in your prayers. God knows the right course for my life, and I will go forward with that assurance no matter what the future holds.

<><

Karen

2

December 4, 2012
Discussing Treatment Options

Hi folks,

Most of you received the initial news last week, though a few of you may not yet be in the loop. Last Monday, November 26, I received the results of a lung biopsy that I had done on November 21. The results were positive for lung cancer. On Tuesday, November 27, I met my oncologist, Dr. Ray, for the first time. He wanted to gather additional information from blood tests and a PET scan (done last Thursday midday), as well as through direct consultation with the pathologist who had provided the biopsy results. The original CT scan that led to this biopsy had showed spots on both my right lung and my liver.

Here are some of the things I learned at today's follow-up visit with the doctor, and also a few things I learned through my own research as I prepared for the visit. PET scans are used about 90% of the time to determine cancer staging and to observe whether the cancer cells have spread to additional sites throughout the body. In my case, it appears that it has not spread to numerous locations, but it has spread to the liver. When I asked what stage it is, Dr. Ray said "by definition, it is stage 4." Please do not misunderstand. That does not mean I am on death's door, but it does mean that it has metastasized, and that it is currently deemed inoperable.

My research has taught me that lung cancer surgery is fairly rare in any case, but there are a number of other treatment possibilities. Before I explain the two likeliest treatment regimens for me, let me mention that the doctor has asked me to get two more tests done (both of which I've scheduled for this Thursday, Dec. 6). One is a bone scan, and the other is a brain MRI. [According to MedicineNet.com: *An MRI (or magnetic resonance imaging) scan is a radiology technique that uses magnetism, radio waves, and a computer to produce images of body structures....The image and resolution produced by MRI is quite detailed and can detect tiny changes of structures within the body.*] This is to double-check and make sure that the cancer has not spread to these locations. I feel confident that we'll get good results on these tests, but in the end...only time will tell.

Now, to explain a little bit more about treatment possibilities in my case...we will not be able to map this out until my appointment next Tuesday afternoon following the additional tests. However, if some test results we are still awaiting prove to be EGFR+, then I will have two options. [According to MedicineNet.com: *A protein called the epidermal growth factor receptor (EGFR) is important in promoting the division of cells. This protein is found at abnormally high levels on the surface of some types of cancer cells, including many cases of non-small cell lung cancer.*] Both are daily oral drug treatments. One is called Tarceva. The other is in clinical trials, but has proven to be even more effective so far than Tarceva. It is called Dacomitinib. Both have only mild potential side effects of rash and diarrhea. I am hopeful that this will be my result primarily because the treatment for this is the easiest one. If the results are EGFR-, I would be in for chemotherapy treatments done intravenously every three weeks. That would be a combination of Carboplatin/Taxol + Avastin, and it would, of course, mean the likelihood of experiencing some of the side-effects that we all hear about such as loss of hair and some nausea. The doctor indicated that the chemotherapy done for lung cancer does not tend to have as much of a nausea side-effect as breast cancer patients often experience with their treatments, however.

After roughly 2 months of whatever treatment I end up doing, I'll be sent back to the radiologist to get repeat scans done to hopefully see significant shrinkage of the tumors. If this continues to be the case after several months, Dr. Ray says we might discuss some aggressive surgical therapy to resection the lung and liver. The way I took this, though we did not talk in depth about it today yet, is that if we reach this point, this could potentially cut out the remaining cancer in me. Of course, everyone knows that the best efforts in this way can and often do leave behind cancer cells that return to cause problems at later dates. Still, this sounds like a promising possibility to me, and because I am still considered a young gal and a lifelong non-smoker, I could potentially be a good candidate.

So, take away from my brief report that I feel relatively good about the outcome of today's appointment. We know what and where it is (though we are still doing a couple of tests to make certain it is not "also" in the bones or brain), and there are some courses of treatment that don't sound too scary with regard to awful side-effects. None of the drug treatments will likely cause me to need to change my daily life routine very much, including my ability to continue working. There may be a possibility of surgery for me down the line a piece, and I believe that would be a positive development if we get to that point.

Finally, I want to again thank everyone reading this for your outpouring of concern and prayers on my behalf. I am always grateful. I know now and always that God goes before me and will guide my way through this to whatever end result is right. I accept that and am happy to be preparing to move forward. Please, again, feel free to share this with anyone who knows me or who you believe should know what I am sharing.

<><

Karen

3

December 11, 2012
Negative EGFR Means Chemo Coming

Hi folks,

This is the first mailing in what may be many to come over time as I embark on this journey to fight off the lung cancer which has taken up residence in my right lung and liver. With regard to emails going back and forth, I hope those of you who feel inclined will not hesitate to reply to my emails and have a bit of correspondence with me. I'm sure there are bound to be some rougher days ahead in this battle I'm facing, so your notes would be encouragement for me to simply keep up the good fight knowing my friends are at my side.

So, today's visit with my oncologist was the third visit I've had with him so far. Now, all the preliminary tests we needed to do have been completed and results assembled. I mentioned that I was to have a bone scan and brain MRI to determine if the cancer had spread to those locations or not. The results were negative on both counts, and that is very good news. The brain MRI did show some anomalies within some blood vessels, but they are not aneurysms, so even though there is history of stroke in my family, my doctor, in consultation with other oncologists on staff at this large cancer clinic, feel that it will be safe to still use one of the drugs, Avastin, that is paired with other drugs I'll be given. More on that in a moment.

I also mentioned that we were awaiting the results of the EGFR test. It would be determinative regarding which direction my treatment would take: daily oral drugs with only mild side effects…or intravenous chemotherapy every 21 days with hair loss and potential nausea and related side effects that are generally controllable with anti-nausea drugs, etc. I was, of course, hoping for a positive result, which would have set me on the oral drug path. But…I got a negative result, which now sets me on a chemo-therapy path. Tomorrow morning, I will speak with Dr. Ray's nurse to begin arranging the various appointments I will need to get everything rolling within the next week on that course of treatment. I'll be given Carboplatin/Taxol + Avastin. Avastin is the drug that the doctors consulted with each other about when told of the stroke history in my family (my mother and grandfather). They feel confident that it will not present a problem in my treat-ment, but I will research it further on my own yet tonight to see if I have any questions that I feel the need to pursue when I speak with the nurse tomorrow morning.

So…as I've told some of my friends, I will soon (it turns out probably within 2-3 weeks, I believe) be losing my hair. This will save me blow drying time in the mornings and allow that little bit of extra sleep. Woohoo!! And, I'm planning to wear a Nationals' baseball helmet as my head covering of choice. Seriously though, I already have a prescription for a wig if I decide to fill it, and I'll probably pick up some nice scarves and have someone show me how to tie and wear them properly. It'll probably be at least 3-4 months minimum that I'm gonna look like Yul Brynner. Wonder if I could get a sweet deal on Broadway during this time?

So, this is really the only news to provide for this evening. Until I speak with the nurse tomorrow morning, I won't know the specifics of my upcoming schedule, but I will pass that along so you can be kept in the loop and lifting me up in prayer with specifics to go on. Although I sometimes try to add a little levity to the situation, I am well aware that it is a very serious matter, and I never take your concern or support for granted.

One final thing for this message…most of you know that my mother passed away last Friday morning, Dec. 7, 2012, and I want to thank so many of you who sent condolences to my family and me. We had a memorial service this past Sunday and were able to celebrate her life with friends and relatives at that time. She was a wonderful woman who is now able to live in the eternal realm with no more pain and physical hardship. For that, I am truly thankful.

I will provide a further update soon regarding my upcoming treatments.

<><

Karen

4

December 18, 2012
Chemo Class Prep

Hi folks,

I chose to wait until this evening to send another update because, following my doctor visit last week, I scheduled quite a few upcoming medical appointments, first of which was my chemo class this morning. I thought that would provide me some valuable information to pass along to you, even though I found it a bit overwhelming. See, I can admit that it's not all as easy or stress-free as I often attempt to make it seem.

Anyway, to get this update rolling, I'll give you the upcoming chemo treatment schedule that is on the calendar so far. I begin this Thursday, Dec. 20. Twenty-one days later (Jan. 10, 2013) I'll have the second treatment...and 21 days after that (Jan. 31), still another. Three days before each treatment, I will go in for lab tests and a visit with my doctor or his nurse practitioner to make sure all of my blood counts and iron readings and things of that nature have recovered sufficiently to undergo the next chemo session.

For me, each treatment will last around 6 ½ hours, so I'll be there all day long and be taking a lunch with me. Lovely setting for a picnic, eh? The start of treatment will consist of being given a course of anti-nausea and steroid medication, and I believe in my case Benadryl to ward off rashes that can develop during treatment. Then, I will be given slow and consecutive intravenous courses of Taxol, Carboplatin and Avastin, though I think they use the generic names which are a lot longer and harder to pronounce. These cannot be given concurrently, and must be in a specified order. So, I plan to take a laptop computer and avail myself of the WiFi there. YouTube can keep me occupied for hours at a time. I'll also have a book on hand, and with any luck, I might even take a nap, however unlikely that seems to me now.

I've already gotten a prescription for a cranial prosthesis (i.e., wig), and also two anti-nausea oral drugs (Compazine and Ativan – trade names) to take the moment I feel the first sensation of nausea starting when I'm at home. I haven't checked out wigs yet, but am told that the American Cancer Society will provide one free each calendar year. Thus, if I get one before Dec. 31, 2012, I could get another in January 2013, I believe. This would allow me some variety, if I choose to avail myself of this once my hair is gone. That event should occur 2-3 weeks after the initial treatment, so probably in the first or second week of January. The nurse who taught this morning's class said for patients receiving types of chemo that produce hair loss, there will be little warning. Once it starts to go, it only takes 2-3 days. Whew!

I've already picked up the anti-nausea drugs and am trying to supply my pantry and refrigerator as well with all the things I may need to take me through this first treatment cycle. For instance, this afternoon, I went out and purchased more liquid refreshments than I think I've ever bought at one time in my life. I will need to keep myself far more hydrated than is my normal pattern. This being the case, I know that I need flavored drinks and will have to push myself in this area.

I'll need to take my temperature each afternoon to make sure I am not running any fevers of 100.5 or higher. Anything above that warrants an immediate call for medical aid because it indicates an infection has set in. This is always a concern while undergoing chemotherapy because white blood cells will be significantly reduced and therefore cannot fight off attacks on the immune system as readily as normal.

As you might imagine, there are plenty of potential side-effects, but I am quite certain it is unlikely that most will occur. Fortunately, there are treatments for most all of them, though too low a red blood cell count or platelet count (it must be VERY low) can require appropriate transfusions.

Because the corticosteroid I'll be given (Dexamethasone), like all steroids, will likely boost my energy level, there tends to be a significant drop off in the few days following treatment. Most patients experience tiredness and on occasion a bit of what is sometimes called brain fog. This, like all of the side effects, may or may not happen to me, but once I see how my body reacts to the first round of chemo treatment, it is likely to react in a similar fashion with each subsequent treatment cycle. That is good to know, because I will be able to plan accordingly after this first one.

Many of you have asked if there is anything you can do for me, or how you can help. Once I get through this first treatment, I will have a much firmer grip on what to expect in the months ahead, and this will give me a better idea of how to answer your questions or offers in this regard. I may need some help walking my dog Bella on treatment days and the few days afterward. I may need drivers to help get me to and from appointments sometimes (though it's possible I'll be able to drive myself if the drowsiness side effects don't hit me as they do some). I may welcome some soups (more liquids) or other foods being offered on occasion. I will be sure to let you know about any of these things, or others that may become more pressing.

Most of all, I will ALWAYS welcome your continued prayers. And unless I am feeling poorly at a given time, I will certainly welcome your communications through email, Facebook, telephone, or even drop-in visits from time to time. I anticipate continuing to work as much as possible throughout this journey, but for obvious reasons, will need to take some days off along the way. I am very thankful that my bosses at my company are being so extremely gracious in working with me to make this battle as easy and successful as possible.

<><

Karen

5

December 20, 2012
First Chemo Day Experience

Hi folks,

Today, as you know, was my first chemotherapy day. Some of you have been through this procedure yourselves or are close to family members or friends who have had this experience. For every person, it is at least slightly different because the drug combinations are individually determined, the delivery manner can be different (many people have "ports" for intravenous drug treatments, but so far, I do not), and everyone's body, mind and spirit react differently to these things. So, I can only tell you how it is for me.

My appointment was scheduled to begin at 9 a.m. this morning, and the clinic staff were quite timely about that. The first half hour or so involved being injected with Benadryl and Pepcid to ward off potential rashes that the chemo drugs can cause. Because everything was done intravenously, the effects happened very, very quickly. Within just a couple of minutes, my eyes began to blur, and I began to feel slightly queasy and very, very tired. I had been reading the closed captioning on a TV screen and also texting with a friend. That had to stop at that point, and my eyes needed to close. Except when I had to verify the accuracy of my name, birth date, and the particular drug to be given, and also when I had to visit the restroom (they also keep constant fluids pumping into one's body during these procedures, so that naturally goes through and back out again), I literally slept through almost the entire Taxol segment of today's treatment. That was a 3-hour long injection. Sleeping would have been much harder without the Benadryl because the stuffed chairs are comfortable and have foot rests, but do not recline much at all. I generally find it hard to sleep sitting up…ask any of my airline travel partners.

The delivery of the second drug, Carboplatin, took one hour, and immediately following that, the Avastin took only 30 minutes. So, that totals about 5 hours when the preliminary meds are included, and with a bit of time in between when my nurse for the day was attending to one of her other patients, the total time I spent at the chemo clinic was about 6 hours.

I left about 3 p.m. feeling very groggy still, but no other real ill effects so far. I have drugs on hand to address possible side effects that could occur in the next few days, so we shall see how things go. I'm hoping for little or no need to address such issues, but only time will tell. Now, at least, we are underway, and I'm glad that is the case. I'm also glad to be learning the ropes so I will not have open-ended questions lingering anymore on some of the matters that every first-time-chemo-patient surely experiences.

I'm just hanging out here at home this evening, doing a few odds and ends, trying to give Bella a short walk to no avail. Hopefully, our neighbor, who took her out at lunch time had more success on that. She just wanted to come back inside with me this evening, and I can tell you that I'm not too disheartened by that tonight. I'm also getting ready to make some supper, force myself to keep drinking stuff, and maybe write another letter if I don't nod off before I accomplish that. If that happens, I'll get at it tomorrow.

It looks like I'll be scheduling my next series of three chemo treatments for February and March when I attend my next treatment day on January 10, 2013. By that time, I will likely look like some of the other ladies who were in attendance today. I think I may suggest we form a Kojak fan club. I could pass out lollipops as a club-warming gift, but maybe one of you dessert type cooks would like to offer me a recipe for such a candy that would be low in sugar (?).

This is perhaps not a super interesting update, but I thought you might like to know how my first treatment day went, so there you have it.

<><

Karen

6

December 30, 2012
Side Effects?

Hi folks,

It's me again. I was afraid you might have forgotten me since it's been a week and a half since my last real update. So, I thought perhaps you would be interested in hearing how I'm doing following that first chemo treatment on December 20.

You already heard about the treatment itself, so the biggest, best news I can tell you is that I have experienced NO nausea side effects at all. That was the one side effect possibility that had me a bit nervous going in, so I am extremely thankful for this turn of events. The first night after treatment, I did as the nurses had repeatedly said to do…at the very first sign of stomach trouble, take an anti-nausea pill. I awoke in the night and my stomach didn't feel nauseous, but there were some minor rumblings, so I took a pill. I'm not sure if that is why I felt slightly light-headed the following day or not, but I had no other ill effects from the pill or from my stomach. That was really the only issue, other than some remaining tiredness, that I felt that first day following treatment.

Some of the physical symptoms I've dealt with since are definitely chemo side effects, and others I am not so sure about. For instance, starting the second day after and continuing for the next few days, I had fairly severe earaches and sore throat, but don't know if I would have had them without the chemo anyway. Eventually, they went away, but I was pretty uncomfortable for the weekend. A few nights after treatment, I awoke in the middle of the night with a nosebleed. That was a side effect. But, I only have had one and it wasn't too hard to correct.

The one significant side effect I continue to face that started 3 or 4 days after treatment day has been neuropathy in both hands and most especially in my thumbs and index fingers. I have it to a lesser degree in both the soles of my feet and my toes. It feels like my fingers are in a constant state of being anesthetized with Novocain that is starting to wear off. You know, that pin prickly, tingly unpleasant sensation? It's the best way I can describe it. But, though there is some numbness, my fingers are not entirely numb, and I can certainly function quite normally.

I inquired with the nurse I contact with questions and was told to try taking B Complex and B6 vitamins. She said that patients with this issue often experience some relief from it with these vitamins. I've been taking a B Complex horse-sized pill each morning now for about five days, so far to no noticeable effect. I did not add a B6 only because the B Complex already has 5,000 daily units of B6 in it. That seemed like a lot to me. So, I'll continue with the B Complex and ask the doctor when I see him on January 7 if I'm doing the right dosage or should add a separate B6 to the mix. I'm trying to avoid having them prescribe Neurontin for me to address this issue because I simply don't want to take more prescription drugs than necessary.

Each day, I take my temperature in the afternoon just to make sure it is staying within normal ranges. For me, it has always been low rather than high in this first round, between 96.2 and 98 so far. That's good. As long as we don't hit 100.5, we're good to go.

One other persistent problem I've had for what seems like weeks now is laryngitis. I am not sure if this is chemo related or not, for my voice was acting a little funny even before the treatment, but has been consistently bad since. Just yesterday and today, it has seemed to have more parts of the day where it is getting close to normal again, but it still goes in and out. It is not painful, but just sounds high and raspy much of the time.

Last week, I went in to work Wednesday through Friday. Due to the holiday timeframe, there was little to do, but it was a good test for me to see how my energy would hold up. Things seemed basically fine. So, this week, I am scheduled to work all but New Year's Day when, of course, the company will be closed. I arranged with the folks who deal with medical leave at my company, based on my doctor's recommendation/agreement, to be authorized intermittent medical leave while I am receiving chemo treatments. I expect to take the treatment day and possibly one or two days following it (with a weekend thrown into that period too) to get through the initial tiredness, but otherwise, I should mostly only need to take off for medical appointments if this treatment cycle becomes the model for all subsequent ones.

This coming Wednesday afternoon, I do have a wig appointment at one of the American Cancer Society locations. I wanted to get that accomplished while I still have hair, so we can try to match my shade and texture as closely as possible. Based on what I've been told, I anticipate that my hair will probably go within the next week to week and a half. While I've been prepping for this eventuality, which my doctor tells me is a certainty with the drugs I'm receiving, I know it will initially be quite a shock to me. I have decided, however, that once it begins to come out, I'm going to be proactive and get my head shaved right away rather than wait the few days it could take to come out in clumps. That just seems worse.

One of my sisters has kindly made me 11 head scarves of varying colors, based especially on my appreciation for primary colors. A couple of friends have given me scarves as gifts. And you may see me occasionally wearing a little beanie cap that my sister-in-law made for my mother. I like it and if you see me wearing something with the name Gerry on its front, you'll know I'm honoring my mother that day (though I hope I do every day).

So, I guess that's enough for this update. Many thanks for your ongoing support. More to come soon.
<><
Karen

7

January 2, 2013
Going for My First Wig

Hi folks,

This is the wig update. Having never set foot in a wig shop, or considered purchasing such an item in the past, I had no idea what to expect. Didn't know if I might surprise myself and want to try some varied colors and styles that would give me a very different look. Didn't know if there would be lots and lots to look at, or only a few. Didn't know if it would take an hour, or only a few minutes. Didn't have a clue what a wig would feel like on my head. Didn't know if they would be made of real hair or synthetic fibers.

Now I have answers to all those questions, and I am going to proceed to bore you ...er share them with you. First, I suppose I should reaffirm that for this first wig appointment, I went to the nearest American Cancer Society location rather than a shop dedicated solely to the provision of wigs for its clients. So, that, and the fact that they provide one for free to cancer patients, probably helps to answer the fact that they were all made of synthetic fibers, which is less expensive. The available selection was not huge either.

I decided right out of the starting blocks that I wanted to try and get something reasonably similar to my own hair color and in a style close to something I either have worn or would be likely to wear. That gave me just three real possibilities in a shade that is a little bit lighter than my hair with probably just a bit more red tint than I have. Still, it's fairly close. I also tried one darker brown model and thought it looked, shall we say, horrid. We took one or two others down for me to look at and I promptly rejected them out of hand. I was a bit disappointed that there weren't any Ann Burrell (look her up) wigs there because I really did want to try one of those! Ah well...

Anyway, as soon as I walked into the wig room, I was given one of those little nylon stocking things to put over my hair (such as it is at the moment), and then we set about the trials. All three of the chestnut/ginger colored wigs looked reasonably okay. They were in varying lengths and I ended up choosing the middle length, which is a little bit shorter than my current hair style. I liked the shorter one reasonably well, but it seemed more of a summer style, so I ended up rejecting it. The one I selected has some mild wave to it which, as most of you know, I like to have in my hair, so that works.

The attendant told me when I asked if these wigs could be styled that heat cannot be applied to them. Thus, curling irons, blow dryers, etc. are out. In fact, she said they should not even be worn in the kitchen while cooking because the bangs could change their color or texture or something. Ah well...they're free, so I guess one can't be too picky, eh?

Now, here's what the few of you on this list who have worn wigs, or know people who have, can probably attest to. The inside of the wigs feel like they are made of burlap. It is a somewhat scratchy open weave material and even with a thin skull cap under it, I suspect I will agree with what I've heard others say, that "it just feels itchy." I am glad, however, that I'm giving myself a variety of options for the days ahead.

I could have led off with this, but why do the obvious? My hair is, indeed, beginning to come out. But, because I've been blessed with thick hair, people don't notice it too much so far, so I'm going to give it a little longer. I can feel it beginning to thin and certainly I see quite a lot coming out in my hairbrush and also on the collar of my winter jacket. While I showered this morning, I very gingerly moved my hands through my hair as I washed it, trying to make sure I didn't rub it all off in the shower! I say that with a smile and an exclamation, but I am mostly serious.

So, all the foregoing said, I imagine many of you might like to see pictures. I am going to disappoint you on that count tonight. You all know what I look like and how I look right now. I'll post pictures once the hair is gone and I can model scarves, hats, a wig, or a bald head. All with a smile. How about that?

One of my friends shared an interesting little wig story with me that even included a photo. If you have any you'd like to share, I'd love to hear 'em. Go ahead…make me laugh.

<><

Karen

8

January 10, 2013

Laryngitis, Neuropathy, and Itching, Oh My

Hi folks,

Today was chemo treatment day number two. As I mentioned in one of my previous updates, I had an appointment to go in and get some lab tests and have a follow-up with the doctor three days ahead, which was this past Monday. All of my lab results were within proper ranges, so on that count, we were good to go. Following that very brief introduction to our meeting, the doctor and I simply discussed how I had responded to the first round.

I mentioned the various side effects or other physical occurrences that I had any questions about, and the doctor offered explanations or ideas as to cause and effect. For instance, I told him about the earaches and sore throat I had developed on days 2-4 following that first treatment. He told me he did not think that was likely related to the chemo. So, I will watch to see what happens in that same period this time. If it does not recur, I will assume that it was indeed simply a little cold of sorts that had set in briefly. If it does recur, I may think we've discovered a new side effect.

I told the doctor about my continuing mild neuropathy in my fingers and also, I told him I was taking B Complex pills based on his nurse's advice, but that it was not making too much difference. He told me I could take a second tablet each day, but that they often don't see dramatic effects from the B Complex. So, at least I now know that I should not necessarily expect much more improvement regarding that little issue for a while. It's always better to at least know these things rather than to have constant questions about it.

When I mentioned the ongoing laryngitis, my nurse in today's chemo session told me that she has often seen chemo patients deal with laryngitis issues. So, perhaps it is not necessarily a side effect of chemo, but it is apparently not that uncommon among some cancer patients. I suspect it will simply continue for some time to come. Neither Dr. Ray nor the infusion nurse offered any ideas on ways to resolve the problem. Fortunately, I am not sick, so to speak, so beyond my voice sounding funny, it really is not a big problem at all.

The one thing I'd forgotten to mention to the doctor on Monday was a creeping development of itching around my body, but particularly on the backs of my hands, my underarms, the balls of my feet, and my lower back. It got rather severe on Monday evening and continued for the next couple of days. I contacted my nurse navigator and was told to come back into the office for a visit with the

Physician Assistant on Tuesday morning. I tried her suggested remedies, which didn't seem to help too much and I must admit I was pretty uncomfortable until today when I got all the intravenous Benadryl and Dexamethasone. I suspect those drugs helped a lot since they are given especially to ward off rashes that often can develop while chemo drugs are being delivered into the body. I just hope the severity of the itching will not return now.

Today, a friend from my church served as my driver to and from the chemo appointment. Because I learned the first time that the preliminary drugs literally knock me out, this was a necessity. The day was similar to the first treatment day, except the drugs didn't knock me for quite as big a loop this time around. I wondered if perhaps my body had simply adjusted to them a little bit. That's not to say they didn't make me drowsy, because they did…and I still slept for a good portion of the 5 ½ to 6 hours that I was there. I like that fact, because it makes the day go by much quicker than it might otherwise. Most of the other patients seem to be getting shorter treatments than I do. Some, in fact, only seem to be there for 30 minutes or an hour. Some are there for a couple of hours. But, of course, they may also be coming back in for treatments on a more frequent basis. As I mentioned in a previous update, everyone has individualized regimens based on the very specific nature of their disease, stage, and the like.

I dined on a cheese sandwich, wheat thin crackers, and some pecan tarts. And, you know what else? I found that the chairs actually do recline a bit. I just had to push in the correct way. That was good to know and made it more comfortable to sleep.

At one point, late in the treatment period, I was getting up from my chair for a restroom call and decided to remove the neck pillow from around my neck before I moved away from my chair. As I did this simple act of putting my hand at the back of the pillow to remove it, I also brought with it a handful of hair. Yesterday and today, the hair is beginning to come out very rapidly, particularly at the back of my head and around the bottom. The top seems to be a bit slower, but I fully expect to finish this job of hair removal before the weekend is over. So...to all of my work colleagues, be forewarned, next Monday will probably be the day for quite an appearance change.

Oh, I should mention that I also was able to take up a couple more friends on their generous offers to help in whatever ways I might need. One, who has served as a long-term pet sitter for me on a number of occasions when I've been traveling, came over to provide a pee break for Bella at lunchtime. Another kindly came over after work to give her a walk. We all expected that I would be pretty groggy following the treatment, as I was the first time. To my surprise, I was not nearly as drowsy this time, so I walked along with them. Then, in the evening, I enjoyed trying out two of the three different soups another friend had made for me. More liquid nourishment that is good for me.

So many people have offered help in whatever ways I might need, and I am very grateful for their efforts and the kindnesses of everyone who is trying to share thoughts, prayers, and assistance as I venture through this new journey. One of the things I enjoy most is the corre-

27

spondence many of you send to me following these updates. So, please keep them coming. And I'll keep the updates flowing all along the way.

<><

Karen

9

January 14, 2013
Bald and Beautiful

Hi folks,

I'm three days into the new bald and beautiful look. Well, it's taken me about three days to reach the beautiful part in my own mind, for as you might imagine, it's quite an adjustment.

My hair had been shedding, so to speak, for more than a week, and for the last three days or so before I made the final call in a very significant way. Every brush stroke through it came out full of hair. Though it never came out in clumps, it had thinned by probably two thirds of its normal thickness before I felt that bald spots would have revealed themselves in only another day or so. There was no reason to delay things any longer.

I had asked my sister Jo to keep her electric hair trimmer in her car so she could simply stop by after work on whichever day I made the fateful call. That call went out on Friday, January 11. She came over that afternoon, I fixed supper for us, and we warmed me up with a little Michael Crawford video viewing. Then, I laid a sheet on the floor, positioned a chair, and sat for the big event.

Have any of you who are not bald ever thought about what it would feel like? I had not, so I guess I would say I was surprised to find that immediately, even while my hair was still being shaved off, my head felt much cooler and sort of damp. There was a lot of hair on the floor, which was testament to the fact that even in its thinned state, I had a lot of it. Following the shaving, I promptly went to my mirror, figuring I may as well just get used to it. I can't say I liked what I saw. Jo told me my head was shaped pretty nicely, and surprisingly to me at least, others who I have let see my bald head so far have expressed those same sentiments. I did not know what my head would look like hairless. It could have had unexpected ridges or boney outcroppings.

The first night, and the second, I slept with a little jersey hat on my head. It kept me warm, but didn't feel very comfortable. Last night, the third night, I decided to sleep without the hat. That was much better.

On Saturday, my first full day without hair, I had planned an outing with a young Ethiopian friend and Jo. I chose to wear a red head scarf on this first day out and about with my new look. First, we took a luncheon cruise on the Potomac on the Spirit of Washington. We went over to the Air and Space museum after that. Most of you know me well enough to know that energy could be my middle name, so we met up with my friend Brad and headed up to National Cathedral for a quick self-guided tour, then off to the zoo for a walk. By that time, it was growing dark, so we headed to our homes. Jo came with me and we walked my dog Bella, then went out to eat and off to a few stores.

This is where I can tell you that I am continuing to learn new things as I move along this journey. The lesson I learned that evening, after about 10 solid hours on the go, was that my energy level is not what I am used to. I began feeling pretty low before we finished our final outings and have needed both Sunday and to some extent even today to recoup from overdoing things on Saturday. I know now that I must pull back a little more, even if I start out feeling good.

Over the past few days, since the last chemo treatment this past Thursday, Jan. 10, the neuropathy is increasing in my hands, feet and even to some degree in my tongue. I

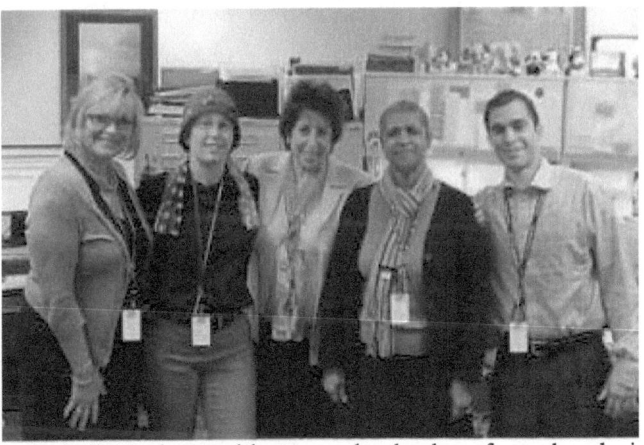

now believe the problem on the backs of my hands is related to the neuropathy. While it itches and is very uncomfortable at times, it still has the pin prickly kind of feel associated with it. The soles of my feet kick up with extreme itching especially when I've been on them for a while. I try to relieve the itching to some degree by placing my feet on an ice pack, and I'll do the same with my hands when I am done typing this. I will also contact my nurse navigator about this to see if there may be any other solutions that could be of help.

I stopped the B Complex vitamins last Thursday because I learned that the Niacin in them could be helping to cause the itching I'd been experiencing. Since then, my back, underarms and stomach have been much better, so I think that may have helped on that count, though possibly the increased neuropathy is related to stopping the B Complex as well. It's a bit of a trial and error kind of thing to find what will work best for this, I believe. I'm still very thankful that I'm not dealing with nausea.

Today, I went back to work and chose to wear a red knit hat with an ornamental scarf woven through it; a thoughtful gift given to me by a friend in Pennsylvania.

This solo shot shows how I look with the free American Cancer Society wig on. I think it looks reasonably nice, though I believe it would itch quite a lot if I tried to wear it for any extended period. I don't know what the future holds for wig usage. Time will tell.

Finally, I chose my buddies Nick and Trent for a nice threesome of baldies. We look good together, don't we? Although, lookout for the glare atop my head!

I may just run with the au naturel look before too long. But first, I need to reach that point where I'm comfortable enough with this new look to rock it out in public. That may not be far off, although it is still winter after all, so it'll be a day by day thing.

<>

Karen

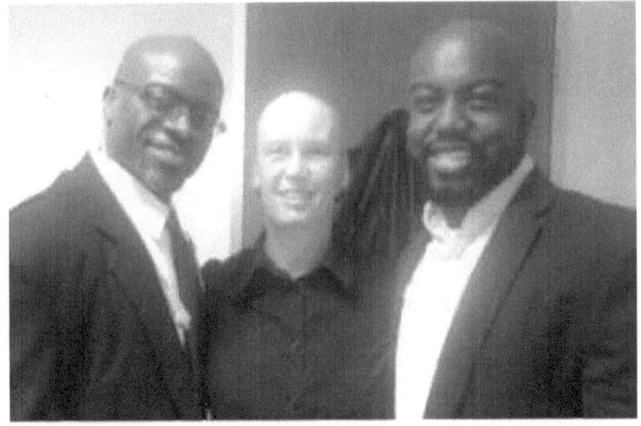

10

January 22, 2013
More on Side Effects

Hi folks,

Since many of you have told me you are finding it interesting to learn of my experiences on this cancer journey, I thought I'd tell you a bit about a couple of side effects I've been continuing to deal with since chemo treatments have been underway. Remember, I'm not afraid to talk about these things, so you may be "in for it" on occasion.

I just returned from my first weekend foray out of town since my cancer diagnosis late in November 2012. I joined my sister and we went to see my father and other sister in Pennsylvania. There is a lot of flu going around, not to mention the common cold, so I try to be cautious about being too close to others who may be sick, and wash my hands frequently as well. In fact, that has played a part in my frequent evening attacks of the hand itchiness. I've mentioned it before, so you surely recall that the neuropathy I've been experiencing is most pronounced in my hands and fingers.

I have come to the conclusion that the hand and foot itchiness, in all likelihood, is related to the neuropathy. The backs of my hands, and sometimes between my fingers, can get very irritated, though still without an accompanying rash. Warm water seems to help set this off, if it is not already underway. So, mealtime can be rough since I have my hands in warm water often as I prepare foods and then do cleanup following the preparation and the meal itself. I feel the pin prickly sensations along with a need to rub my hands because they itch. Of course, the more I rub them, the more they itch. It becomes a cycle. I try to resist rubbing them as much as possible, because I know it will get worse.

Last evening, a friend brought me some salve which is not unlike petroleum jelly. I was under attack when she arrived, so I lathered up with the stuff, so to speak. This was after I had already run my hands under ice cold water for 30 to 60 seconds to dampen the discomfort. The itchiness did reduce in intensity to where I could leave it alone, but I don't know for sure if the salve made the difference, or the water did, or a combination of the two. My friend also brought some specialized soaps and body washes that we hope may aid me in trying to deal with this ongoing issue. These were very thoughtful gifts and I appreciate them.

As for my feet, the itchiness mainly comes around the balls of my feet. It is quite intense when it happens, and it seems to be a very, very quick onset. It causes me to want to remove my shoes and rub my feet over a rough carpet. The easiest way for me to try to relieve some of the itchiness in these instances is to place my feet on an ice pack, or to gradually stop the rubbing as much as I am able until it eventually calms down.

These attacks seem to happen most often in the evening, although when I went to Pennsylvania, they happened while I was driving. Since it is winter, and cold besides, I was able to place one hand directly on the window and drive one-handed. This helped a fair amount. It was like using an ice pack on my left hand.

As for the other side effect that I promised for this message…well…we're going to get down and dirty! Maybe you guessed it…we're talking constipation and hemorrhoids. You know those unpleasant, unfortunate, uncomfortable, unmentionables. But we're going to talk about them here.

Late last summer, I had my baseline colonoscopy. I learned that I had no polyps and was basically in good shape down there, but I do have some internal hemorrhoids. Well, I could have told the doc that before she found them. Now, as I deal with chemotherapy and the side effects that often come along with it, including constipation, which I've been "lucky" enough to experience, I find that the hemorrhoids are not just internal, but also external. Perhaps more of you reading this can understand or relate to this issue than the cancer itself. Anyway, they hurt, particularly when I am using that part of my physical makeup (see, I still have a sense of decorum about how I describe things).

Initially, I just worked through the days, eating more fiber, trying to drink more fluids than I am used to, and the like. But, after the second chemo treatment, this problem seemed to grow and with it the hemorrhoid problems also worsened. So, I contacted my nurse navigator. Well, I contacted her about this AND the ongoing itching problems.

After the nurse consulted with Dr. Ray, she replied to me and told me the doctor had called in a prescription for Lyrica, a drug to combat the neuropathy. I would take 50 mg a day for 3 days, then 100 mg a day for three days, and finally reach a dosage of 150 mg a day. So far, I am not noticing any significant difference from the Lyrica, but will continue the 150 mg dosage, which I just reached today, and hope it just takes a little more time before the effects of the drug will kick in with positive results.

As for the constipation issues, I was told to buy Colace over the counter and use it as needed. I have done exactly that, and continue to try and enhance the fiber in my diet and the fluids as well. The hemorrhoids still bother me a bit, but I am healed enough that things are better for now, thankfully.

So, aren't you glad we had this little communication? Next time, I may talk about mucus or phlegm!

<><

Karen

11

January 29, 2013

Impacts on Friends and Loved Ones

Hi folks,

This is going to be a little different than past updates in some ways. I don't have much of anything particularly new to report on the medical front. I guess I can tell you that at my labs and follow-up visit yesterday afternoon I confirmed that the chemo side-effects do, indeed, tend to be cumulative. That causes me to be a little unsettled considering that I've had such discomfort with the itching on my hands and feet related to the ongoing neuropathy. Will it get still worse with treatment number three, then four, five and six? I surely hope not, but time will tell.

As it is now, when my hands "kick up," it is hard to settle them down for hours afterward, though I continue to try, mostly with ice packs or ice cold water. And I continue taking the Lyrica at 150 mg per day, but may raise that to 200 mg per day in another week if need be, per instructions of the physician assistant I met with yesterday. I add a Benadryl tablet to that before bed each evening, but since it knocks me out, I only take it at nighttime. So, if you want to know something specific to pray for related to my experience, I would ask you to pray that the itching would cease.

Today, I thought I'd write a little bit about how this journey I'm on impacts people in different ways. Or, perhaps better put, people can choose to respond to it in different ways. Some may become depressed about the size of the challenge, feeling that it is a mountain too high to climb. The side-effects are too great. After all, who wants to lose her hair? Who wants to have numb hands and feet? Who wants to lose her sense of taste? Who wants to feel sicker during treatment than before it began?

Others may pull away from relationships for reasons they may or may not understand. Possibly, they believe they are trying to make things easier for loved ones by staying away or reducing contact because they believe it will only make others sad. This may or may not be the case, of course, for every person in every relationship reacts in his or her own way.

Still others may try to pretend the medical problem does not exist, even though they may be going through serious treatments to deal with it. They won't talk about it. They will do everything possible to hide what is happening because it may be too scary for them to contemplate. They may know the statistics related to the disease, and particularly if those stats are pretty ugly, to put it bluntly, they may choose to force them into a deep, dark place in their minds, and tightly shut and lock the door over top of them.

But there is another way some may deal with a disease like mine: metastatic lung cancer. It is the path I've chosen. That is to consciously make a firm determination to maintain a positive outlook and attitude, not only for those looking in from the outside, but for myself too. As a 16-year survivor of uterine and ovarian cancers, I chose when I learned of that diagnosis to do everything in my power to conduct myself in a way that I hoped would be inspirational to others. When I received the diagnosis of metastatic lung cancer late last November, my determination was even stronger, IF possible, to do the same this time around. I'm not trying to win plaudits from others, but I want to "let my light so shine among men" that others will see Jesus through me. In fact, perhaps I was put on earth just for this. Do you ever think about these things in your own lives?

So far, I feel very fortunate that I am not experiencing many severe side-effects from the treatment I am receiving. I am able to continue working, and that in itself is a blessing. But, I know that the real possibility exists that things could get significantly rougher for me in the weeks and months to come. Right now, it is not so hard to stay upbeat, but if I end up being physically beaten down at some point, things will be much more difficult. It will be at that time when the mental strength and determination will really come into play. It will be at that time that I will need to pull from a strength that is not my own, a strength that is aided by you who are reading this, but much more from my Lord and Savior who walks by my side and will carry me when I can no longer walk on my own.

I suppose that's enough of the serious stuff for this message, but from time to time, it's important to let you know that I don't shy away from the harder parts of this experience. I must deal with it, and learn about it, and face it head on. Even while I'm doing exactly that, I figure since I have lost my hair, I may as well have fun with it. Right now, I have enough head attire, mostly given to me by others, to take me through at least four weeks without repeating a single day.

With that in mind, I'm including a photo you may enjoy of one of the more fun looks I've been sporting lately. See if you think it suits me, or am I completely jumping off the deep end with my best imitation of Frank Spencer from the 70s British sitcom *Some Mothers Do 'Ave 'Em.*

<><

Karen

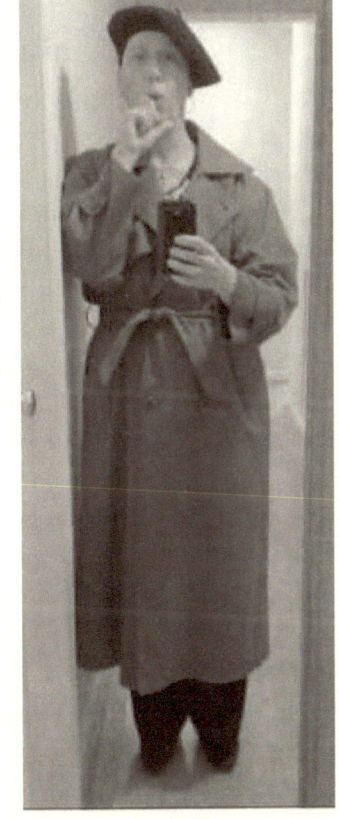

12

February 2, 2013
Halfway Through

Hi folks,

I completed chemo treatment number three this past Thursday. I am now halfway through my scheduled treatments. Woohoo! I've gone ahead and scheduled a PET scan for February 15, per my doctor's orders, just a few days ahead of treatment number four. On the prescription, it is called a re-staging PET/CT scan, but in reality, I don't expect it to restage the cancer. What we do hope to see is a reduction in the size of the tumors in my lung and liver. If that continues to happen through the entire chemo process, we may be able to look to therapies that will give me a better prognosis for the long-term future.

Many of you may be wondering how the itching is doing now, nearly a week since I last wrote about it. Well, I believe the nurse who served me on Thursday was probably rather surprised when I told her I was glad to be there and eager to get the pre-chemo drugs going. You see, I get slammed with Benadryl and Dexamethasone, among other drugs, before they begin the chemo drugs. This is to ward off nausea, rashes, and other potential side effects that sometimes occur during the delivery of the chemo drugs. For me, however, it seems that those two drugs, in particular, may help to ward off the neuropathic itching for a while too. So, I felt pretty good on Thursday and Friday, and even today I'm doing okay. As long as I keep my hands away from warm water, and resist rubbing them, I'm managing pretty well. The Benadryl did cause me to sleep for the entire 5 ½ hours of treatment, except for the short period I awoke and ate the lunch I'd brought with me. The nurse assured me, when I asked, that I did not snore while I slept. That would be a little bit embarrassing when there are so many other people present, so I was glad for the assurance.

All of you know by now that I have been hairless for about three weeks now. But, what you may not realize is that when chemotherapy causes a person to lose his or her hair, this does not just happen on top of the head. The chemo drugs are not able to zero in on cancer cells alone. They go after all fast growing cells in the body, and hair follicles, fingernails and toenails are some of the other cells that get killed off by these harsh chemicals. So, I don't know if you have noticed in some of the photos I've attached to recent updates, but while I still have eyebrows and eyelashes, they are beginning to thin considerably.

Some of the blog posts I've read from other cancer patients make clear that the eyebrows and eyelashes tend to be about the last to go, and often don't depart until the end of the chemo treatment period. But, when they do go, many people find this to be the hardest hair to lose because it is what makes a person truly look sick. It takes features away from one's face. As I looked at some of my recent photos, I noticed this becoming evident with me with the thinning of my eyebrows, so I decided it was time to get signed up with Look Good, Feel Better, a class provided through the American Cancer Society. At these classes, an instructor helps cancer patients (classes are for women or men, but not both in the same class) learn to apply makeup in ways that will help them to look good and feel better about themselves. Supplies are given to each student to take home and use. For me, I am looking forward to learning how to apply eye makeup to my advantage, because even during the best of times, I tend to look like a raccoon when I make such attempts. So, I'll attend this class on February 11, after which time I'll report back to let you know what I learned. If it turns out well, I may even include some pictorial evidence to prove it.

Tomorrow is Super Bowl Sunday. I have lost much of the excitement I once had for professional football, but like most red-blooded Americans, I'll be watching the big game anyway. This time, for local proximity reasons, I'll be rooting for the Baltimore Ravens and sharing the experience with my sister. We'll have our own little party with the following menu: hamburger barbeque, fried eggplant, broccoli/cauliflower salad, deviled egg potato salad, and of course, tortilla chips and salsa. For me…this is the end of a sports season that has more import to me because it means BASEBALL SEASON IS ALMOST

UPON US. Now that is something I can get excited about.

Thank you all for your continued support and communications with me following each of these updates. I enjoy hearing from you and appreciate your warm words of encouragement.

<><

Karen

13

Some Days ARE Hard

Hi folks,

In my effort to be honest about this journey I'm on, and to share the experience with all of you, I am going to let you know in this update about some harder parts of dealing with the whole thing.

I gave myself a few days to regroup before writing this update, and am now beginning to think that days three and four following treatments are going to be my worst days. After the first treatment, I had severe earaches and a sore throat on those days. Treatment number two brought some mild queasiness and severe itching on those days. But, on days three and four after treatment three (this past Sunday and Monday), I felt absolutely miserable. I slept very fitfully both nights, felt somewhat queasy, though not entirely nauseous, had severe shortness of breath at times that caused my panting to the extent that I had to lie down momentarily to recover my breath. The neuropathy became even more noticeable in my tongue and lips, which in turn seemed to be taking my taste sensations away.

While these various side effects were going on, the neuropathy in my hands and feet continued unabated with the accompanying itching that has been a seemingly unending source of discomfort for at least a month now. I had run out of Lyrica on Saturday and my pharmacy would not refill it initially because they claimed it was not yet time according to my doctor's orders. This was incorrect, since I'd been following those orders exactly. Nevertheless, there was a two-day lapse in my Lyrica doses. I continue to be uncertain about whether it is making any difference in the neuropathy problem anyway. I believe it "may" be helping to keep it at a certain plateau level, rather than actually helping to take it away. On the other hand, I am beginning to believe the Benadryl is possibly aiding me more in keeping things in check enough on the itching front that I can usually resist scratching.

Because Benadryl puts me to sleep, I take an adult dose before bedtime, and have begun, just yesterday, taking half a dose (a children's dose) at lunchtime to try and tamp things down for the evening. This really is a trial and error process, even for the doctors who attempt to help their patients deal successfully with side effects.

So, with regard to all the foregoing about days three and four, I not only felt miserable physically, I will tell you that my brain and soul were feeling very stressed as well. As much as I try to stay positive as I move through this part of my life, from time to time, I have no choice but to let my guard down. It takes work and energy to fight on, to smile through adversity, to maintain that determination I talked about in a previous update.

Many of you will understand when I tell you about some communications I had near lunchtime on Monday that were helpful to me at just the time I needed help. You see, I had come to work Monday morning, though I probably should not have. I struggled to do some work that had accrued over the weekend, and told my supervisors that I needed to go home and would do so very soon. Every time I tried to wrap things up so I could depart, more work came in that needed to be undertaken that day. My job as a meeting coordinator deals with much activity that is highly time sensitive. Anyway, I found that the morning hours had come and gone as I continued working away, still feeling unwell.

Just before I left for lunch, I logged into Facebook and told a friend about my woes. She asked if there was anything she could do from afar (she lives in Chicagoland). I told her the best thing was that she allowed me simply to complain…to let out some feelings of upset. Then, I went home for lunch still feeling highly stressed. While there, I logged back into Facebook where I am able to communicate with so many friends from distant places. As luck would have it, a good friend from New Jersey was online. I began a brief chat with her and before long she decided we needed to talk by telephone.

After I explained that I simply felt highly stressed to the point where it was leaking out of my eyes and down my cheeks, she told me it was okay to feel that way. Folks, I am smart and I understand all of that, but by nature I am stoic. That is my comfort zone, but in this instance, I simply needed a supportive friend to verbally tell me it was okay. That helped me release the stress, get back on track, and regroup to fight on. I guess this update is intended to let you all know that sometimes all it takes to help someone is a listening ear and a kind word of support.

Friends from my company came over and walked Bella on Monday after work, and I took Benadryl a bit later and zonked out for a long and peaceful sleep through the night. I awoke Tuesday morning feeling much, much better, and have continued through the week without further incident.

I will now expect days three and four to be rough in subsequent treatment cycles, and this in itself will help me prepare my mind for what's to come. Knowing that day five will almost certainly bring relief and point me into a generally good continuation of the cycle can only help. So, I look to the future, treatments four through six, with optimism. Just as I am trying to impart knowledge to you who are reading this, I continue to gain wisdom as I move through this journey. So you see, even old people are capable of learning!

The next update will provide information on my ACS makeup class. There is a good possibility this could be quite comical. Stay tuned.

<><

Karen

14

February 13, 2013
Taking a Makeup Class for Cancer Patients

Hi folks,

Before we get under way with this update, I wanted to tell you about my new nickname. My name, as you know, does not lend itself to nicknames as a general rule, so I never really had one growing up. There was one friend who occasionally would call me K-K, but that seemed a little too juvenile for me at this point in life, so I had to deliberate for a time. You know, get the old imagination juices flowing. Unfortunately, I suppose I wasn't super creative with the outcome that I finally chose. It took me back to my childhood and Walt Disney's feature length cartoon movies. Many of you will certainly remember Snow White and her seven dwarfs, Grumpy, Dopey, Doc, Sleepy, Sneezy, Happy and Bashful. Well, the theme seemed right to me, so I've decided to …have you guessed yet…become…Itchy. Yes, that's the ticket. The theme ran with descriptive names, so I'm going with it. You may feel free to call me Itchy from now until I tell you to stop. By the way, I would LOVE to tell you to stop very soon. I'm just sayin'.

Now then, back to the business at hand. I went to Look Good, Feel Better class this past Monday evening. I figured I would be well advised to learn how to draw on eyebrows once mine depart completely. They've actually lightened to a sort of blonde shade as they have thinned, so I guess I'm getting a little bit of a feel for the look already, even though I still have them.

Anyway, it turned out that the class was indeed designed to provide makeup tips, as well as products. The kits that were handed out to each of the five of us attending were labeled light, medium and dark. As the instructor went around determining what each person needed, she got to me and, in a very quick delivery, said "light". Turns out, I have a light complexion. Who knew?! Even so, my kit had a foundation so dark that I could never use it, even if I get a tan, or what almost passes for one on me, ever again. So, I gave it away before the evening was out.

Then, everyone else there proceeded to methodically take up each new product and apply it to her face. Well, that was after we'd all taken one of the damp towelettes provided in the kit to clean our faces of any makeup that might be on them. I did so with the towelettes provided in my kit and immediately turned candy apple red. Then I promptly began to break out. Ah…the memories of youth. I don't believe I'll be using any more of those towelettes.

Everyone began applying the concealer, then the under eye cream to remove dark semi-circles, the foundation, the powder, the eyeliner, the eye shadow, the mascara, the eyebrow pencil, the lip liner, and finally the lipstick. It's very possible I've forgotten something.

Wow! I have never been well versed in makeup applications. Now I know why. I think I've kept myself looking reasonably nice through the years, but I'd say I use about four of those products to produce my "look". Now, I only wanted to learn what to do with missing eyebrows and eyelashes. We didn't address the latter, but I did get a good tip for the former. I was told to consider purchasing an eyebrow stencil. I apparently have "classically" shaped eyebrows. In the American Cancer Society booklet we were given, they are called "Allure". Then, I just need a soft brown eyebrow pencil and practice. I can use a little brush on them once they are drawn in, if I choose. Since I still have thin brows, I'm not ready to practice on my face yet, but I know how to measure where they should be, so I won't have them half-way up my forehead or something rather unusual like that.

I had told the instructor that she probably should know that I would be far and away the most inept person in the class. I mean, how are you supposed to adequately apply a carefully drawn eye line when you can't see much of anything without your glasses on? Well, I suppose I could draw it on top of my glasses lenses. Now there's an idea! As time went on, and the instructor realized that she would have to spend most of her time with one special needs student, she came up with a plan. I told her I had once studied oil painting, so she looked through her materials and came up with a visual aid for me. She told me to look it over carefully, then taped it to the side of my mirror and suggested I try to duplicate it on my face. Some people questioned my truthfulness about this part of the story. Well, in all honesty, it was the only paragraph where I did take some liberties.

In the end, I came home with a nice little makeup kit, some of which I might actually use, most of which I probably won't. But, the idea was a good one and I did get some worthwhile pointers.

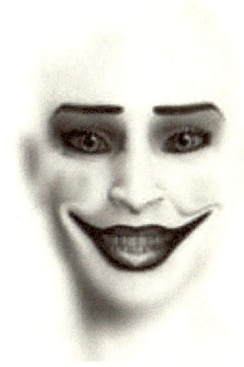

Now, on to a completely different topic. This Friday morning, February 15, I will have a repeat PET scan performed. This will tell my doctor and me if the chemotherapy is having the desired effect – shrinkage of the tumors. I don't expect to know the results until early next week when I go for an appointment with my doctor following my pre-chemo labs on Tuesday. So, it would be nice if you would pray for a very good outcome of this PET scan. You might also be interested to know that the laryngitis I've had for more than 2 ½ months now seems to be lessening. At least, I have more short periods where my voice is "almost" returning to normal. If it has been due to the lung tumor pressing on the laryngeal nerve, as my doctor believes is the possible culprit, then this also seems like it may be a hopeful sign that things are improving inside of me.

Many thanks for your ongoing concern, support in so many ways and communications.

<><

Karen

15

February 23, 2013
Mid-Term PET Scan Results

Hi folks,

I've been planning to write this update since Tuesday evening, but I've been tired or involved in other activities and simply haven't gotten around to it until now. So, I hope those of you who have been waiting with baited breath will now breathe just a bit easier.

In fact, one of the points of this particular update is to tell you the results of my "midterm" PET scan, which you will recall was taken last Friday, February 15. The simple answer is that both tumors, in the lower right lung and the liver, have begun to shrink. My understanding of the report indicates that the nodule on the right lung base has decreased from 2.8 centimeters to 2.1 centimeters, and "there is interval non-visualization of previous foci of increased uptake in liver." So, I cannot tell you a lot about the liver tumor, but Dr. Ray told me both were decreasing, so that's the objective and it is a good result.

Yesterday, I had my 4th chemotherapy treatment. As usual, it went well and took 6 hours. The neuropathy continues, as does the related itching, though that has been fairly mild yesterday and today. It seems to cycle around and I do get a day here and there where it is not too bad. I am very thankful for those days of respite.

Last weekend, I was invited up to my aunt's church in Marysville, PA to hear one of the songs I wrote performed as a part of the morning service. It is the same song I used as the soundtrack for the video slide show tribute we used at my mother's recent memorial service. A good friend helped with the arrangement. I based the chorus on my mother's favorite Bible verse, Philippians 4:13, "I can do all things through Christ who strengthens me."

Opportunities like that help to continually keep my spirits uplifted. In fact, Thursday evening, another friend came over and helped me by performing a few maintenance needs in my two bathrooms. His wife sent over a Mexican style casserole. I am very grateful for such acts of kindness. Just the day before, another friend took me to one of our favorite restaurants for a lovely dinner and time to visit with each other.

While people are doing these nice things for me because they want to help me while I am battling this challenging disease called metastatic lung cancer, I hope we will all continue to show love and kindness toward one another…even in the good times. This experience brings out the goodness in so many people who I didn't even know cared about me before. Maybe they didn't even know it either…but now we do. How wonderful is that?

Oh, and I must tell you one more hugely important

thing. Last week on Thursday, Valentine's Day, one of my supervisors called me in the morning and asked me to come to his office. I didn't know what he wanted but told him I'd be right down. So, I stepped into his office and he handed me a bag with a Washington Nationals' baseball helmet inside, with these appropriate words…"Happy Valentine's Day!" That man knows the way to a gal's heart! Seriously, he remembered that I'd said my head covering of choice during this period of my life was going to be a Nationals' baseball helmet, only I had not found one so far. Being one of my best baseball buddies, he took it to heart and went out and found me one. And I wore it all that day in the office. And I will wear it again. It will see plenty of use.

<><

Karen

Christis My Strength (song and lyrics by Karen Loss)

I've lived through dips and troughs of life.
When days were tough, and full of strife.
At those dark times I prayed to God,
Recalled the journey Jesus trod.

I can do all things because Christ strengthens me.

When life was rough, my heart felt fear.
I cried to God, "Incline your ear."
He said, "I sent my Son for you.
Look to Him, he'll see you through."

I can do all things because Christ strengthens me.

My voice back then was very weak,
But now no longer spent and meek.
Each day I laugh and smile and sing
Because Christ is my everything.

I can do all things because Christ strengthens me.

My savior said that love is all.
With faith and hope, I will not fall.
I've seen the light of love on earth,
Yet long for heaven's eternal birth.

I can do all things because Christ strengthens me.

When my life story is complete,
I'll rest in knowing who I'll meet.
My heart will sigh and bid adieu,
When Jesus says, "I've come for you."

I can do all things because Christ strengthens me.

I'll take His hand and walk with Him
Assured His love will never dim.
My God has said to have no fear,
For His own Son is ever near.

I can do all things because Christ strengthens me.

16

March 3, 2013
Michael Crawford and Doggy Snuggles

Hi folks,

I hope you have not forgotten me since I last wrote many eons ago, or so it seems. I didn't want to write with nothing of any significance or interest to tell you, so I waited. I hope it was worth it.

First, waaaaaaaaaaaaaay back on February 19, while I was waiting in an examining room for my follow-up appointment prior to chemo treatment number four, I received a call on my cell phone. Perhaps I should back up just a bit and tell you that I am huge Michael Crawford fan. He is the actor/singer who originated the title role in Andrew Lloyd Weber's <u>Phantom of the Opera</u> stage production. I had the good fortune to see him as the phantom in Los Angeles during his final run in 1991, and then again in concert here in Washington, DC in 1998. Well, I've been secretly smitten all these years and finally, though I had resisted for 20 odd years, I joined his international fan association about a year ago. Michael had required that those who wanted to form the fan association in 1991 make it a charitable endeavor, devoting much of their efforts and proceeds to children's charities that he supports. In fact, he has been president of the Sick Children's Trust in England since 1987. It is very similar to Ronald McDonald House. It is one of the things I admire about him.

After I missed out on the first 21 years of member only events, Michael meet and greets, and preferred seating at many of his concerts and stage shows, I thought I'd better get onboard before he stops performing and decides to retire. It seems I may have gotten in near the tail end, or at least during a time when he has chosen to slow down his performing schedule in a major way, so although I've made many good friends in the association during this past year, none of them is named Michael. But then, an opportunity came up -- one that I simply couldn't resist. There would be a raffle, entries of which were gotten by donating to any of the charities Michael supports. That was an easy call on my part since I share his interests in many of these charities. The four winners would receive what, to me, is a first-rate prize. We would get to spend an afternoon with Michael, getting to know him, share stories with him, laugh with him, and who knows…maybe even getting him to sing to us.

Here's why I am telling you this lead-in story. While I've been battling this lung cancer you've been reading about for a few months now, different people have told me, in an honorable sense, that as long as I've got to deal with cancer, I should use it to my advantage where I can.

Now, I don't know if the cancer is why I became one of the four selected winners of this great prize (Woohoo, Yippee, Hurray and all that kind of stuff!), but I did try to put myself in a position to be a "set-aside" winner even if I were not a "legitimately drawn" winner. You see, I wrote Michael himself two letters after I knew of my diagnosis telling him briefly what I was facing, and that I would be so thrilled if I were to meet him in March. Well, more accurately, I also let him know that I was rather certain he would be terribly saddened if he missed out on meeting me in March. I also gently let the association bigwigs know how much I was hoping to win and that, as I fight this medical battle, it would be so great to spend some time with Michael.

When I received the fateful call on February 19 in the doctor's office from the fan association executive director, here is the brief conversation that took place. She told me I was a winner. I responded, "Oh boy, I've been praying for that." Her response was, "Everyone wanted you to win." I was happy to hear that, thought it sounded as though it may, or may not have been a legitimately drawn win, and didn't care. I took the express elevator up to cloud nine at that moment, and haven't fully come down since. So, this may have happened without the cancer, but I'm not at all sure of that, and I believe it belongs in my cancer journey memoirs.

Here's another small tidbit that I haven't mentioned previously, but think many of you might find interesting. Most of you know I have a little American Cocker Spaniel named Bella. She's a cute little dog who likes to snuggle at night. She used to belong to my friend Ernesto, whom many of you have been praying for due to his recent brain cancer diagnosis. Because of his international performing schedule and need to be away from home so often, he sought to find a new home for Bella when she was approaching three years of age. By then, she was already well set in her ways including her insistence that she would sleep on the bed with me. This turned out not to be much of a problem; she is very good about quietly settling in for the night. She simply lies down and goes to sleep, although she does tend to end up tight against my neck before morning.

I am not sure if it is significant or not that Bella has, in just the past couple of months, decided not to sleep on top of the comforter on my bed as she had always done before. Now, she has decided that as soon as the lights are turned off, she'll burrow in beside me…right under the covers. Still, she settles in and calmly goes to sleep. Now, as you may have noted, her timing, and my cancer battle have coincided fairly closely. It makes me wonder if she has sensed what I'm dealing with and this is her canine way of getting even closer to me just now, maybe to help heal me in the best way she knows how. I certainly think it's possible. What about you?

<><

Karen

17

March 10, 2013
Itching to the Max and Hand Healing

Hi folks,

I can say, with great thankfulness, I am writing to you in a physical state that is MUCH better than it was for several days this past week. You see, last Sunday, I ran out of Lyrica, the drug I'd been prescribed for the neuropathy. My prescription had no refill on it, so I could not call for the pharmacy to get one. But, the fact is, I wasn't at all sure it was helping me anyway since, as you know, I've continued to have problems with itching and it didn't seem to be improving. So, Monday morning, I contacted my nurse navigator and asked if it was okay to simply go off of the Lyrica, at least until my appointment with Dr. Ray the following Tuesday when we could reevaluate the matter, if necessary. She responded that it was up to me and if I wanted to go off of it, that was fine.

As a result of that communication, I thought I'd find

out if I was indeed correct, that I had been taking a drug that I did not need…or if another thought I'd had might be correct. Was the Lyrica actually helping to keep the itching from being even worse, even if it was not eliminating the problem? It didn't take long for me to begin to have a pretty good idea which answer was the correct one. Right away on Monday I began to have more intense itching. Tuesday and Wednesday were even worse, and Thursday was the worst of all. By Wednesday, the day being hyped as Snowquester here in the Washington, DC area due to the forecasted storm that barely even made its presence known, I contacted my nurse navigator again and said, "Please call in a new Lyrica prescription…NOW!!!"

I'd been sitting at my desk with my feet on ice, periodically running to our floor's pantry to run icy cold water over my hands, and feeling as uncomfortable as can be due to the intense itching. It was also bothering my buttocks and the backs of my legs, for they too felt the friction of the seats I would sit on just to work at my computer or do other normal tasks of the day. Naturally, when I went to the pharmacy to pick up my prescription, they said, "Oh, we're out of that today. It won't be in until after 4 p.m. tomorrow." Through gritted teeth and slits for eyes I confirmed the statement I'd just heard and said, "I need it…I really need it."

So, I sucked it up, took a double dose of Benadryl to help me get through the night, and awaited late afternoon on Thursday when I could get my new Lyrica prescription. By 4:30 p.m. that day, I took a dose and a half of the Lyrica, 150 mg. It seemed to begin helping fairly quickly, but that might have been because, to my surprise, it really started to knock me out. I had not noticed a drowsiness side effect to it before, but then I had never taken that much at one time. Since I became so tired, I found myself lying on the couch with my feet up, dozing through the evening. It helped to keep my feet up and not feel the friction of shoes or floors from walking.

By Friday morning, with another regular dose under my belt, I went to work feeling quite a bit better than I had all week. It was good to find out whether or not I needed the Lyrica, because I really don't want to put more drugs into my system than I truly need. In this case, the answer is now definitive, and I am thankful for that.

When a person goes through a journey like the one I'm taking, I believe it is imperative to not only research the disease and its standard treatment protocols, but also to consider and contemplate the use of complementary treatments that appear to have good potential for helping to eradicate the disease. You see, my goal is to not only accept the fact that I have metastatic lung cancer with its challenging odds for long-term survival, but to do what I can to beat those odds. American medicine directs my treatment to chemotherapy, and then potentially other therapies including surgery to try and remove the disease from my body. I have embarked on this path and you have been reading all about it. But I've learned of other complementary treatments that I believe may also help me.

One such treatment was brought to my attention by a good friend whose work colleague has her Hungarian father-in-law visiting for a few weeks. It turns out he is a hand healer who feels he has been gifted by God to heal people. I agreed to see him since, although I knew nothing about his technique, I felt it could not harm me and might potentially help me. His technique sounds much like Reiki. Anyway, mostly he does not touch me, but moves his hands very closely over my body. He does lay his hands on the middle of my right back right where the lung tumor was biopsied. And he lays his hands on my front mid/lower right roughly where the liver would be. He slowly and gently rotates his fingers clockwise in those two areas for several minutes.

After several of the Hungarian hand healers treatments, he has made the claim that the lung tumor is gone. I don't yet know if he is right. It'll take another PET or CT scan to tell that for sure, but I actually think there is a good possibility it is, indeed, gone. My laryngitis was persistent for literally three entire months, and about a week ago, it began to depart from me. My voice is now back to its normal dulcet sound. Okay, perhaps not dulcet, but still normal. That definitely indicates something good.

Oh, one more thing I wanted to tell you in this update…just another way that God continues to bless me only because He can. You know that I am traveling to southern California this month and will, during my stay there, meet Michael Crawford. Well, I needed to find someone who could give me a lift to the airport very early in the morning on March 19. After church today, I stopped to talk to a friend and, out of the blue, she asked me if I needed a ride to the airport because she'd be happy to give me a lift. I had not even raised the subject with her, but gladly accepted her offer. I long ago stopped believing in coincidence, because I have so often seen God answer these seemingly small and insignificant needs which sometimes end up in my prayers, but not always. So I hope you will all join me in a "Yay God!" shout out. I look to him for everything, and I try to glorify His holy name through the life I live. I hope you do too.

Thanks again to everyone who is reading this, caring for me through your prayers, thoughts, gifts, and friendship. I love reading your correspondence, so keep it coming. It warms my heart.

<><

Karen

18

March 18, 2013
Adding Herbal Treatments to My Regimen

Hi folks,

I'm getting a quick update off to you all before I pack it in for the night. I have an early morning trip out to Dulles Airport to get started on my little vacation to southern California that will finish up with my Michael Crawford adventure. I'm looking forward to it, but I'm looking even more forward to a good night's sleep and hopefully as itch-free a week as possible. Then, I can concentrate better on what lies ahead.

For this update, I have a few odds and ends to share with you. First, I thought you might get a kind of weird kick out of a coincidence I realized a week or so ago. Yeah, I know, I told you I don't believe in coincidences. Well…anyway, it turns out that cancer's been a recurrent theme in my life…from the very beginning. You see, even though I was supposed to be a Leo, I wanted out into this big, wide world sooner than planned, so I forced my way out just in time to be a...you guessed it...Cancer. Okay, I know. I sometimes have a sick sense of humor. Get it? Alright, really, enough of that. I can take a good-hearted smack if you feel it necessary.

I decided that this update was the right time to tell you that I have been doing a second "complementary" therapy to go along with the chemotherapy. In addition to the hand healing I told you about in the last update, I've also been following a treatment regimen prescribed for me by a Chinese cancer specialist. I was referred to Dr. H by the doctors at the pain clinic where I've been successfully treated for a shoulder ailment that had troubled me a great deal for more than a decade. I'd seen what seemed like every kind of specialist imaginable for the shoulder ailment, unfortunately, without a correct diagnosis or any noticeable help. Finally, in yet another attempt to get relief from the recurrent shoulder pain, I found Dr. Dave and his associates.

When Dr. Dave repeatedly told me that it might be to my advantage to meet with Dr. H and see if she might be able to treat me for the cancer I'm fighting, I felt it was well worth my while to look into this option. Dr. H has experience in both Chinese and American medicine, though she has chosen to practice Chinese medicine. She specializes in the treatment of cancer of various forms and stages, and her patients have had remarkable success in being freed from this insidious disease.

American medical professionals often are not terribly open to treatments and methodologies from other parts of the world, even though in at least some cases, they may have been shown to be quite successful elsewhere. The argument is frequently that we don't have conclusive studies showing the efficacy of the treatment, or telling them the adverse reactions that could potentially be caused with other drugs they are using in American-style treatments. This was also my cancer clinic's answer when I made an inquiry about adding this complementary therapy to my treatment plan.

If it weren't for the fact that I was referred by American doctors, and that Dr. H is also trained in American medicine and understands the drug/chemo treatment I am receiving, I would probably have taken the advice to not add herbal therapy in my care plan. But, as you can surely tell by now, I decided that in the end, the final decision had to be mine and therefore I've chosen to add this Chinese herbal therapy to my regimen.

Since February 19, I have been drinking four ounces of a strong, unsweetened tea made from eight different herbs, and taking two specially formulated American ginseng capsules twice a day. And this has made a very big difference in my mindset.

You see, from the time I was diagnosed in late November until February 19, I accepted my condition, the treatment course I had set upon, and the very grim statistics that are a part of the Stage 4 lung cancer story. I accepted that I might end up in the very, very small percentage who beat the disease, but realized that the odds were heavily against that outcome. I knew that I could go forward accepting whatever was in store, and that's exactly where my head was. I was doing what I needed to do by American standards to fight the disease, and trying to stay upbeat, but not having any good sense of the final outcome.

Beginning February 19 when I started Dr. H's herbal treatments, my mindset changed. From that day to this, I now believe that I have this disease beaten. I am still realistic, and know that I could be entirely wrong; however, I have an expectation now that I will be cancer free soon. In fact, I can't wait for my next PET or CT scan because I have a strong suspicion that Dr. Ray will be shocked to get the results...but I won't be. If I'm right, I believe they won't show shrinkage in the tumors. I believe that report will read, "No indication of cancer present."

So, you see, it is important for me to have sought the advice of the medical personnel at the cancer clinic, but in the end, I believe it was even more important for me to have made the decision to, in this case, choose not to follow their advice. Time will tell if I've made a wise decision, but it's not just a physical thing. It's a mental and spiritual thing. I'm still completing chemo, as ordered, but I'm adding more firepower to my battle plan.

So, here are a couple of prayer requests I'd like to put before you in this update. Obviously, pray for my various treatment plans (chemo, Chinese herbal therapy, hand healing) to be successful in completely ridding my body of every single cancer cell. Pray that the neuropathy and related itching would decrease and eventually go away entirely (sooner rather than later). Pray that my California trip would be a happy time with few side-effects from this chemo treatment I've been undergoing impeding me along the way.

Finally, you might be interested to know that, in accordance with many of your suggestions to this effect, I've begun putting my updates and related materials into manuscript format for a possible book with a working title of *Trekking Through Cancerland*. Any thoughts about that?

<><

Karen

19

March 27, 2013
Meeting Michael

Hi folks,

I'm back from California and I can tell you, it was a great trip. Six days of fun and a time that allowed me to make many new friends. So, this update may not be heavy on the medical part of the update, though I'll touch a bit on that. It'll be more of a "what I did on my early spring vacation," with the variation of doing it while continuing the fight with cancer and the side effects from its treatment. Remember those reports from elementary school? Or perhaps you've done everything you can to forget them. Well...here goes.

With my sister Jo along on the trip, we flew off to sunny, but rather cool, southern California on Virgin America Airlines. The economy seats were very tightly configured and I couldn't sleep (as usual for me on airplanes), but at least they were leather and the safety video at the start of the trip was funny. We managed to get our rental car soon after we arrived and over the next six days, we put well over 700 miles on it.

One of Jo's friends was kind enough to loan us her home for the first four nights we were there. It was about midway between Los Angeles and San Diego, so we decided to go to the San Diego zoo on day two of our trip. Though both of us had lived in southern California in the 1980s and 1990s, neither of us had ever gone to that zoo, the one that we've always heard is supposed to be one of the best in the country. I was not sure if I could manage all the walking usually required on zoo visits, and considered renting a wheelchair for the day. Once inside, however, I opted to give things a try with the understanding that I would likely need to sit down and get off my feet frequently. If my feet decided they could not take it, we could always ride the bus back to the entrance and get a wheelchair. To my pleasant surprise, I managed to get through the whole 5-hour zoo visit on my own two feet. We even walked in excess of three miles, so I was quite pleased.

Day three required a lot of driving. First, we went up the 405 freeway and into the San Fernando Valley – familiar territory to both of us. We then headed west toward Calabasas and off through the canyons that took us down by Pepperdine University and eventually to Zuma Beach, just north of Malibu. This is the location I generally chose during my infrequent trips to the beach during my time in the Valley. Jo had wanted to stop at a beach for some pictures, and we both decided to go barefoot through the sand and possibly into the edge of the surf.

I remembered that the Pacific Ocean, unlike the Atlantic coast, was always rather frigid. So, I was very surprised to find that when we rolled up our pants and walked into the water, it actually felt pretty good. I went in deeper so that when the surf would roll in it could reach as high as my knees. Again, on this day, I had a very pleasant surprise. My feet felt great while I was in the cool, but not freezing water. We stayed for roughly an hour and a half. Even saw a sea lion pup come up on the beach all by himself, then make his way back out into the surf where he bobbed and played for a while before we finally lost sight of him. What fun!

After we showered the sand off of our legs and feet, we dried our feet, unrolled our pants, put our shoes on, and continued on our way. Next stop...Santa Anita Racetrack over in Arcadia, just past Pasadena. That was a pretty long haul from the beach, so it would be our last touristy kind of stop for the day.

Jo had been there once before, but I'd never been to horse races anywhere and was very interested in going. I love horses and thought it would be great fun. The only problem was, neither of us had a clue how to place bets. So, we figured we'd just watch a few races for the enjoyment of it. I must say, however, on one race, I picked out two horses that, in my mind, I was putting $10 on to win. In reality, I would have too, had I known how. Anyway, sure enough, Red Man Run, one of those horses galloped in to victory at 16:1 odds. Aghhhhhhhhh! Oh well, a good Christian gal like me isn't supposed to gamble anyway, right? I keep telling myself this. It became my internal mantra for the evening.

On day four, we visited one of Jo's good and long-term friends in Orange County then drove up to Long Beach to meet some of the other winners in the Michael Crawford raffle, as well as Coordinating Committee members (CoCos) from his association for dinner at a restaurant on the water. I'd never met any of these folks before, though had had some interactions with them by email. I found them to be lovely people and enjoyed this first meeting very much. In fact, one of the committee ladies was in from Australia (this is an international association), so I made a beeline to sit beside her so I could pick her brain. Some of you know that I've been planning a big trip "down under" for 2014 if my health holds up sufficiently until then. Don't worry, I'm planning that it will. Pat, my new Australian friend, was very accommodating.

When day five, a Saturday, rolled around, Jo and I had decided to join a few of the CoCos and one of the other winners and her daughter to take in the Queen Mary, which has been moored at Long Beach for a few decades now. First we did what any red-blooded American women (or men) would do when they get together. We found the nearest restaurant and we broke bread together. Doesn't that sound better than "we ate 'til we waddled out of there?" Then, we toured the ship, and a new friend and I added a quick tour of a WWII Russian submarine right beside the ship. It was quite fun, but I found my feet beginning to kick up while we did this, so I realized that the few good days I'd had in that regard might be coming to an end.

Upon our return from the Queen Mary, we cleaned up and then headed to O'Malley's Irish pub for dinner with a larger group of CoCos. There, I had a wonderful conversation with the executive director who was giving me the detailed rundown of how she got involved and eventually became the leader of the pack, how the organization and Michael have interacted with each other over time, and just interesting things like that. I was good, as I had been the night before, and had a salad with roasted chicken along with iced tea. I was beginning to get ramped up for the day to come.

Sunday arrived and I posted my song for the day to my Facebook wall. It was Anthony Warlow singing "This is the Moment." Yes, I was headed out to meet and spend a few hours with Michael Crawford on this day. I am going to attach the write-up that I provided to the association for its website rather than write it up here. I do need to say, however, that it was an outstanding experience for me, and when I talked to Michael alone at the end of our time together about my cancer journey, he remarked that he hopes our time together will help me to heal. Well, it surely was good for my soul, and that can only be good, right?

<><

Karen

Write up of Visit with Michael Crawford

First things first...I need to offer a huge thank you and shout-out to Michael for his willingness to share a few hours with me (and the others). Many thanks also to Bobbee and her team of CoCos who all went out of their way to befriend me (I was the newbie of the group) and to show us all a good time leading up to today's fun with Michael.

Now, as to what you all want to hear about, Michael arrived about 5-10 minutes after we did. He said he'd learned about each of us and was quite sure he could pick us out. Then, he proceeded to get each pick wrong as CoCos did their best with hand signals to correct him. It was an act that he'd planned and was cute, indeed. Moments later, we were ushered onto the balcony for photos. Michael was himself from the start, delivering wisecracks and sharing lots of laughter. As we walked back inside to prepare for our departure to the boat with Michael walking ahead, I thought, "Gee, that man, after seven decades, is still fit and trim and doesn't look bad from behind. I must learn his secret!"

Our very capable photographer snapped a few shots

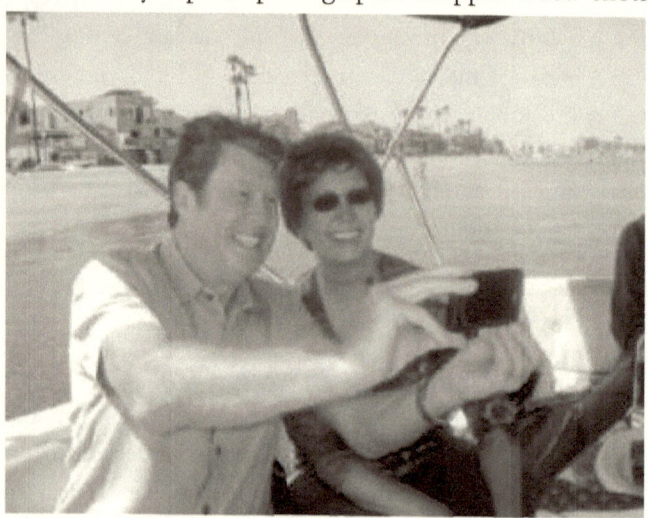

of us at boat side as we were about to board. Then, Michael helped push us off, hopped aboard, and we set about our voyage through the canals and waterways around Long Beach. Over the next couple of hours, we all chatted, often about boats, waterside homes and grandchildren. Downton Abbey even found a way into the conversation for a bit.

We dined on sandwiches, picnic salads, chips and cookies. I purposely waited until Michael had a full mouth of food before asking him myriad questions. Okay, not really, but I did enjoy sitting next to him because it afforded me the easy opportunity to keep tapping his arm and annoying him, er providing conversation starters. He was a perfect gentleman, though I did notice him flinch whenever he would see my right hand begin to move in his direction.

In reality, I had a truly lovely time meeting Michael. As one of the newer (newest?) members of MCIFA, I'd never had the chance to attend a Members Only Event, so the first impression I had as he walked through the door was that he was very down-to-earth and sounded exactly like the guy I've had such fun listening to on YouTube and MCIFA videos. The last impression I had was that I'd been given a wonderful gift by someone who heretofore did not know me, and therefore his generosity that we all know about became very real to me.

Thanks Michael! You're the best!

20

April 4, 2013

It is Finished (Chemo that is)

Hi folks,

My Facebook status update today says simply, "It is finished!" A large percentage of my "friends" on that site know exactly what that means, and I suspect everyone receiving these updates may "get it" too. In case you haven't kept up lately, however, I had my sixth and final chemotherapy treatment today. Like all of the previous ones, I was able to sleep through about two thirds of it. Well, I should probably say, I had no choice but to sleep through about two thirds of it. Those pre-chemo drugs do their trick for me every single time. I get mildly queasy as they begin to take effect, have to close my eyes due to that and intense drowsiness, and before I know it…voilà. I'm sleeping.

Today, my nurse was initially not able to get the IV started properly, so she got a heating pad for me to wrap around my arm for a time. This was to help bring the veins out in a way sufficient to make another attempt that was successful a bit farther up my left arm. It turns out that the veins they use for these intravenous chemo infusions sometimes will never rebuild to their initial size. Apparently, the harsh drugs, particular the Taxol, can cause this. I don't think it will result in any major problem for me down the line though, considering that I have NO PLANS to need more chemotherapy, and hopefully no other frequent needs for intravenous drips either.

I also must take my blood pressure daily for a while now too, because today's reading was the highest it's been during the whole chemo journey. It came in at 160/101. Throughout this chemo period, it's been slightly high, which is unusual for me. My BP has always been considered in the normal to low range. Just as Taxol has been the harshest of the drugs on my veins and is the primary cause for the challenging neuropathy side effects, the third drug I've been receiving, Avastin, is the almost certain culprit for the heightened blood pressure. You may recall my mentioning early on in these updates that my doctor consulted with other doctors in his clinic about my family history of stroke before deciding that the benefits outweighed the risks of including Avastin in my chemo regimen.

Now, these drug infusions are behind me. I can begin to heal naturally again. Woohoo! It will take at least three weeks or more for the chemo drugs to be through my system. After that, my hair will begin to grow back – in what shade or texture, no one yet knows. I'm still keeping my fingers crossed for the platinum blonde Ann Burrell look (You know I'm kidding!). The main thing I'm hoping against is a totally gray or white look. If that were to be the case, I would simply have to alter things in order to maintain my youthful appearance. Can you believe it? A little vanity is creeping in. Anyway, the eyelashes and eyebrows should start coming back within a month now too. That'll be a good thing, because most of you know how much I hate messing with much makeup, and as a result, simply don't let myself care about it enough to make the time and effort. Saves me a lot of money along the way too. I figure, I'll just let my effervescent personality shine to such a degree that no one will notice!

In this past week leading up to today's appointment, I took family friends of a friend of mine on a nighttime Washington, DC memorial tour, and also on a tour of Arlington Cemetery the following morning. We had been messaging back and forth about plans for these tours for several weeks and, as a licensed DC tour guide who is currently on hiatus from official duties, I thought it would be fun just to share time showing some friends around unofficially. As you might imagine, after I made all of these arrangements, there came one of those head slap moments where I said to myself, "Karen...WHAT WERE YOU THINKING? You can barely walk a quarter mile before your feet begin to flare up in a terrible way." Unfortunately, I'm also someone who will NOT go back on my word, once given, if at all possible. So, I did the next best thing. I borrowed a wheelchair from my church, took a friend along to push me, and rode as much or more than I walked. It worked well, and we all had a great time. Solutions to life's problems are usually available if we just open our eyes to the possibilities.

Another thing that has continued to bother me, perhaps more than it bothers my work colleagues, though I can't say that for sure, is that I find it nearly impossible to get myself out of bed at my intended early alarm times in the mornings. As a result, I've been frequently going into work about an hour later than usual. This has caused me to contemplate whether the drugs are simply affecting me so strongly with their sleep inducing measures, or whether I have become lazy and too willing to let myself take advantage of the "poor little ol' me" circumstances that it's easy to sell these days. I'm going with about a 67:33 split on this for now. If, once the chemo is well past, I find that I'm still not forcing myself to get up with the early alarm, I'll know it's the latter. Then, countermeasures will have to be brought to the fore, like a basketball air horn alarm clock, perhaps.

Just last weekend, as I was opening Saturday's mail, I found a card with a return address from the MCIFA. I opened it and found a lovely generic inscription that says, "To our dear friend, Karen. Love from all of us." Then, underneath the Hallmark verse on the right side, it says, "To add my prayers for strength & healing – With love, Michael Crawford XOX" There were three pages of caring and encouraging messages from some of those association members I've come to know best over the past year, and I have since learned that one of my best friends in the association instigated this outpouring of love and support. These types of kindnesses mean more to me than you can possibly imagine. All of you who continue to correspond, pray, network my updates further out to your own prayer groups, and simply care in whatever ways you do…well…I just want you to know you have my undying (get it!) love.

Finally, perhaps the most important thing I have to tell you in this update is that my next PET scan is scheduled for April 22, 2013. I expect to get the results on April 25 when I will have a follow-up with Dr. Ray. I am actually glad that it is that far out yet, for it needs to be near the end of the chemo cycle that just started today. This timing will also allow me to have nearly three more weeks of the Chinese herbal therapy behind me. That will bring me closer to the 10 weeks time Dr. H told me I should plan on before seeing major results from her treatment plan. I am fully expecting good, no, GREAT results in this next scan. And, you all will be among the first to know, either way.

<><

Karen

21

April 11, 2013
Awaiting PET Scan Results
While Wearing New Hats

Hi folks,

Now, we are largely in a holding pattern, flying in circles until we get clearance to land on April 25 when the results come in from the upcoming PET scan. Even though I had my sixth and final chemotherapy treatment one week ago today, I remain in the heart of the three week cycle for that treatment. These cycles tend to happen in patterns where the first couple of days are usually pretty comfortable for me, then days three and four tend to be when I feel a bit queasy, lose my sense of taste temporarily and sometimes develop symptoms similar to an oncoming head cold. Then, we move into the rest of the cycle where the itching resumes its more feverish intensity and the constipation and related hemorrhoids duke it out for supremacy. My body becomes very sensitive all over due to neuropathy, so I am cautious about all forms of touch including how I shower and perform other personal hygiene activities. Sometimes blow dryers with cool air options come in handy even when one has no hair.

I can tell you that this final cycle has followed the normal pattern...except that over time the chemo drugs build up and the side effects become more pronounced. That has been the case with me over the past few months and, this time, I received no respite from the itching those first few days. Darn! I was really looking forward to that too. I lost virtually all of my taste for a couple of days, but didn't really feel too sick overall, so that part was basically good. The rest, well, it continues to follow suit with previous cycles.

The good thing in all of this is that after six rounds of poison being injected into my body in order to try and kill off cancer cells, I am still basically healthy for all intents and purposes. I go to work virtually every day. I attend church most every Sunday. I go out to eat with friends and relatives from time to time. I do almost everything I normally do except walk my dog and guide charter tours around Washington, DC. My feet simply won't stand (or walk) for that right now. Thankfully, I have a friend who is providing this huge and much appreciated dog walking service for me over the past couple of weeks. Bella thanks him too.

Something else happened this past week that came totally out of the blue. Shortly after I arrived at work on Monday morning, four of my colleagues from down the hall came to my office area and presented me with a large bag filled with gifts. They seemed very excited and wanted me to open at least the top item in the bag right then. It turned out to be a pink Washington Nationals baseball cap. Knowing what a huge Nationals fan I am, this was, of course, a very thoughtful gift that they knew would be a big hit. I told them truthfully that it will receive its first wearing tomorrow, April 12, when I attend a game against the Atlanta Braves. Once they'd left and two of my work mates returned to our office, I was told to open everything. They looked on as I opened hat, after hat, after hat…all from different work colleagues, some of whom work in our Massachusetts branch. Over the next two days, I received five more hats to add to dozen given me on Monday.

It turned out that my friends had been conspiring to do this quickly, before my hair begins to grow back, because they had all realized that I'd finally run down my

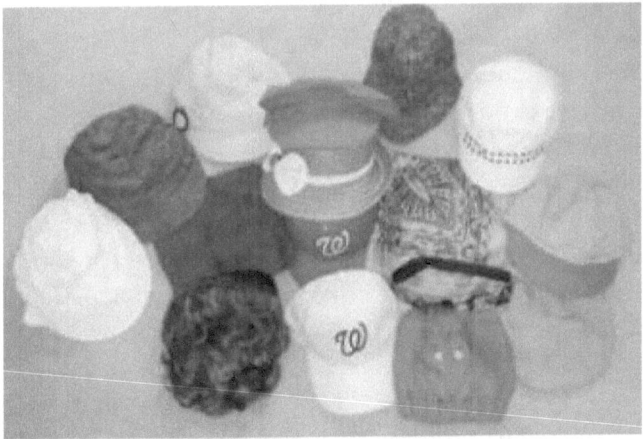

hat, scarf and wig collection to the point where I was beginning to repeat head wear. This could not go on, they reasoned, and so this lovely gift idea came to pass. Now, I'm all set for at least another three weeks of new and varied clothing for atop my bald pate, and I've taken a photograph of most of these new hats so you can enjoy the variety with me.

You'll see that some were taking the warming spring weather into account, even going with white summer styles. Others intentionally went with Nats' red. In any and every event, I love them all because they bring sunshine into my existence. My work colleagues, all of whom are friends, did this out of kindness.

I know I bring that word, kindness, up repeatedly in these updates, and you are likely to continue reading it and other synonymous words in the weeks to come. If it hasn't occurred to you yet, let me emphasize once again that the power of the spirit and the mind are almost certainly the most important part of receiving healing from any disease or serious challenge we face in life. When people treat others, and in this case I happen to be a major recipient, with overt acts of kindness, good things happen to all parties involved. We feel better. We smile more. We laugh louder. We share of ourselves. We learn what it really means to be fully human.

Another thing I bring up frequently is my belief in the power of almighty God to work His will as He sees fit. I also believe that God hears and answers prayer, and through you, and those you share my story with, hundreds, and I believe thousands of people in places all around the world are lifting me up in prayer daily. I hope we all take the time to think about the power that is within all of our grasps to intercede for another. Once we do that, we need to simply know that the final outcome will be right. I am thankful that I know this beyond the shadow of all doubt, and therefore, I can look to the future for whatever it may bring.

<><

Karen

22

April 17, 2013

Hat Stories and Drippy Noses

Hi folks,

To start off with tonight, I must tell you about my experience wearing two of my new pieces of head wear to a recent Washington Nationals baseball game. One item given to me was a new wig. It's not just any wig though. While it is the closest one I have to my real hair color, it is what I call a ¾ wig. You see, it is designed only to be worn with caps or hats. The top of this wig has nothing but air and a couple of elastic straps to help hold it in place. There is only hair around the sides and back to give the illusion of a person with hair when said person has a hat covering the top.

With that introduction, the rest will make more sense. I decided that this wig would be perfect with my new, pink Nats cap last Friday. It is our casual day at work, so I wore this combo all day long and it looked fine. Then, that evening, my buddy and I were going to the Nats game and

I assumed I was all prepped for it with this look that I'd taken on for the previous eight hours already. As we hopped on the Metro train and progressed stop by stop, eventually going underground on our way to the stadium, I was deep in thought. Soon, I turned to my friend and exclaimed, "Oh no!" He looked alarmed and asked me what was the matter? I said slowly, with a sense of dread, "the national anthem." Fortunately, it didn't take long for me to come up with the obvious solution. I would simply go to the bathroom during the national anthem and avoid the need to remove my cap. So that's what I did. And all was well…I thought.

We happily watched our team play solid baseball for

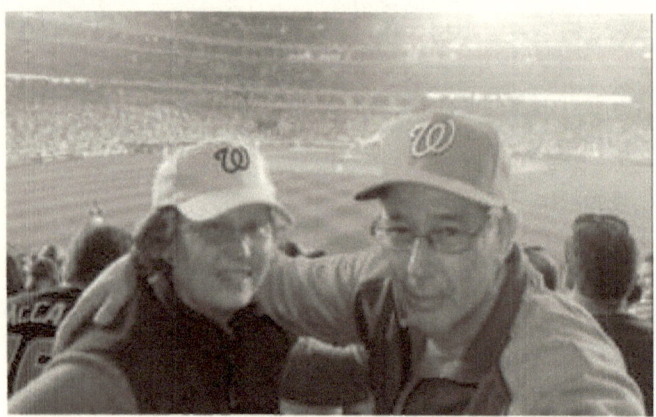

the first 6 ½ innings of the game, and then came the 7th inning stretch. We stood along with all the other fans and prepared to take part in a rousing round of Take Me Out to the Ballgame, only once the music began, I heard a soloist singing God Bless America. Oh no!!! Not again. Every hat in the park, as far as I could see, came off and people stood attentively. I frantically whispered a couple of times that my hat was NOT coming off (even though I felt bad about that). And it didn't. In all my pink-topped glory, I must have stood out to anyone looking on, but it was the way it simply had to be on that occasion.

Finally, we got into the 8th inning and our team's manager had removed the starting pitcher who, up until then, had been pitching a great ball game and had a 4-1 lead. Unfortunately, our relievers, one after another, gave up hit after hit after hit, and eventually a homerun for good measure. At one point, following yet another hit against us, I threw my arms up in frustration and tipped the bill of the cap as I went. It flew off into the air and landed a few seats away on the ground. My head, with the hair around but not topping it, was shown to all who looked on in all its sordid glory until I could scramble about to grab my cap and hurriedly replace it. I guess it was just meant to be on that night. And except for a momentary flash of embarrassment, I found it rather amusing and thought perhaps you would too.

My hat story continued the next night, but in a much different way. I had been invited to a lovely dinner party that had been planned in my honor (and I truly was honored by this act of kindness). Little did my hosts or the other guests know, however, that I had planned, somewhat at the last minute, to bring along the after dinner entertainment. Once we finished a lovely and tasty Mexican themed meal, I showed a few pictures that I hoped would interest everyone at least a little. You know, Michael Crawford with me…and me with Michael Crawford. They smiled and gave sideways glances to one another as I heard little sounds like "Ah" and "Oh" and other vowels. I took that to mean they were loving this. Then, I brought out the hat bag. And a big bag it was. My show was going to reach its zenith with a fashion show.

And so I told a few stories along the way as I tried on various wigs, and numerous hats. I showed and explained about scarves and how they fit, how they are tied, and all sorts of fun or not fun things. My evening audience said they enjoyed this little foray into fashion square. Who would have EVER guessed I would give a fashion show? Anyone?

Now, moving away from hats, I wanted to mention one other thing regarding side effects that heretofore I have not told you about, at least not this part of it. Besides the neuropathy, hair loss, and constipation, you know, the primary side effects I've addressed many times, I've also had a runny nose for months now. Well, I've had this condition ever since the chemo treatments began. Related to it are bloody nose issues, but I've only had two official bloody noses. Otherwise, I simply see blood whenever I blow my nose. But the runniness is what I wanted to address here in this update. It turns out that although I do have some congestion fairly often, and particularly in the mornings, all day long my nose will run, literally with fluid like water. (Brace yourselves. This is that mucus talk I threatened to have in the January 22nd update.)

Anyway, I can be simply sitting at my computer minding my own business, breathing normally, and all of a sudden this water-like substance flows from my nose, literally dripping on anything in its path. I grab for a Kleenex (I don't go anywhere at all, including to bed, without some in my pockets) to blot my nose. And then it stops, until it does it again whenever it pleases. That might be when I'm talking to someone in the hall at work. Or when I'm in the checkout line at the grocery store. Or when I'm watching a ball game at the stadium (had to throw that in). It's not all that troublesome, but can be a bit embarrassing because it happens so quickly that sometimes I can't even reach for a tissue fast enough to blot it before it's dripping.

The last time I was at the chemo infusion center I heard a nurse explain to another patient who was speaking of the same nose problem with her that this happens in this way because when we lose our hair during chemo, as I've noted before, it's not just head hair we lose. It's not just eyebrows and eyelashes. It's not just the hair on our arms. It's also nose hair. Who knew? That had never occurred to me. So there's nothing in this little noggin of mine right now to slow this stuff down. Interesting, isn't it…if we keep our ears open, they're bound to hear new and interesting things all the time. And now, you know my chemo related mucus story.

I'm going to close this update with a reminder that my upcoming PET scan will take place in the morning on April 22nd. That's only a few hours more than four days away. I'll learn the results the afternoon of April 25th. You will know the results that evening too if you check your email. I put together what I hope and believe has been a strong battle plan, and I have followed it conscientiously these past five months. Whatever the final report tells me will lead to the next phase of my life. I will address that further next week when we know those results.

For now…from your lips to God's ears, as the saying goes. But please, don't let it just be a saying, okay?
<><
Karen

23

April 25, 2013
Praise God for Good Results

Hi folks,

ALERT: No humor contained in this update. Good news will have to suffice.

This is going to be one of my shorter updates in recent memory. I don't have a lot of details to provide for now, but expect more to come in about a week when I revisit my doctor following a newly scheduled liver MRI on Monday, April 29, 2013.

My results from the PET scan taken on April 22 showed no sign of the two liver lesions that appeared very bright in the original scan done at the end of November 2012. I did not see the February pictures for comparison today, only the November and April pictures. The upcoming MRI is to make sure there is nothing in the liver that simply isn't lighting up the screen but could still cause trouble. I have learned that even if one test comes up clear, doctors will often run a different test to make sure, because each type of test can bring out different kinds of images and sometimes show existing problems that are not evident in the other test results. It is a good double-check mechanism.

The lung tumor is much smaller and much dimmer in the April 22 scan than it was in the November scan -- also a very good thing. The PET scan pictures were again quite striking in their differences between November and April. This lead Dr. Ray to remark that he's just not quite sure if this is consistent with stage four inoperable lung cancer, and that following the liver MRI next week, he will consult with a thoracic surgeon to get his thoughts on my case based on the various tests and their results. If the liver MRI shows no disease at all, then it sounded like we are probably going to be discussing the possibility of lung surgery to remove the small tumor that still shows up in the most recent scan. Of course, I hope that if it comes to that, by the time we get there and do the pre-surgery pictures, that it too will be 100% gone.

When Dr. Ray first came in to see me today, he said he'd been reviewing the scan pictures and reports and was not quite sure what to think. He was indeed "perplexed". As we talked about this, the reason for his perplexity was due to the fact that what he was seeing is not at all in keeping with the normal progression or expectations for someone with stage four lung cancer. He made reference to that a few separate times. I sat there listening and asking appropriate questions, but also thinking to myself that I was pretty sure I knew why he was seeing these unusual results. I believe a consistently upbeat personal outlook toward my medical circumstances and the prayers of many are changing the course of my cancer trajectory in a very positive way, and science doesn't always know how to deal with that. It made me smile internally and gave me hope for even better things in the future with regard to completely eradicating this disease from my body.

After my MRI, and my doctor's consultation with the thoracic surgeon, we will meet again next Thursday to discuss and consider the best way forward. And I will let you all know what's happening along the way.

Before I close, I simply want to shout "Hallelujah and Praise God Almighty" for His goodness and mercy. I will praise Him when times are good, and also when times are hard. I remain eternally grateful that He has surrounded me with so many loving and supportive friends and relatives. We are all learning important things through my journey, and I love knowing that I can be used for good in this way.

<><

Karen

24

May 2, 2013
Yay…No Evidence of Metabolic Activity

Hi folks,

Your responses to my last update (April 25) were overwhelming. It was like a powerful, yet tame tidal wave rolling in to an empty beach, and then easing back out into the ocean as nature would have it do. Then, I promptly went about losing nearly half of those wonderful and encouraging messages. Seriously though, thank you to so many who forwarded the previously sent ones from the three days following their delivery that were, due to my technological ineptitude, lost in the ether world. As I mentioned in my urgent plea afterward, I've been trying to keep a complete record of my journey through this cancerland, and your messages are certainly a part of that.

Many of you have been wondering, just as I was, what results came from the liver MRI I had this past Monday (April 29, 2013). As with all the previous MRIs I've had, and there have been many, I walked out of the radiology office with a DVD full of pictures. Of course, they are pretty meaningless to the 99.9% of us who don't know how to read them in any useful way. I looked at them and guessed, knowing full well that it was a fruitless waste of time. So, I simply waited for my doctor visit today.

I went to the appointment expecting good results. In fact, what I expected, and obviously wanted, to be told was that there was no sign of disease remaining in my liver. After all, that was what the PET scan appeared to show just last week. Well, my oncologist has been down this road many more times than I have (duh!), so he knew something more might remain in the liver than the PET scan was showing. And that is, indeed, what the MRI was prescribed to evaluate…and what it eventually brought forth. One of the original lesions was "not visualized on this study." So, it duplicated the PET scan in that one lesion is apparently gone. Unfortunately, the second lesion has apparently decreased somewhat in size, but only from 1.5 x 1.4 cm to 2.0 x 1.0 cm.

The PET scan done the previous week (April 22, 2013) gave information from the skull base all the way to the mid thigh. As you already know, it is used primarily as a cancer staging test. The report provided a comparison study with the February 15, 2013 PET scan. The right lower lobe nodule in the lung has "continued [to] decrease in the size and metabolic activity." There is also a "stable tiny 4 mm anterior diaphragmatic node with no metabolic activity." The report also noted "similar mild activity in the posterior right thyroid gland SUV 2, prior study SUV 1.9. No discrete mass." SUV has to do with metabolic activity (or how bright it lights up in the scan). Both the lymph nodes and the thyroid are not considered problematic at this point.

The impression provided by the radiologist indicated "no evidence of metabolically active distant metastatic disease." This concurs with what I wrote in last week's update. It is certainly a good thing. It does not mean the cancer is gone, even in my liver, but it is currently not showing any metabolic activity there. Dr. Ray affirmed again today that he feels these results are very good. He said he had talked with a number of colleagues and has decided to direct me, for now, to what is called Avastin maintenance therapy. This is one of the three drugs I have been receiving since last December when I would go for my chemotherapy treatments. Now, I will continue to receive it every three weeks, but without the other chemo drugs. This one does not have most of the side effects I have written about; however, it has caused my blood pressure to rise to a borderline high level. We will continue to keep an eye on that and potentially may need to medicate for it.

I asked the doctor how long I would need to continue the Avastin maintenance therapy, and he said until the disease begins to assert itself once again. At that point, I will probably be directed to undergo more chemotherapy. He did not feel that major surgery to resection the lung and liver is a great option at this point, and I am relying on his experience to guide me in that regard.

So, although my doctor seemed quite pleased with these results and how well I am doing, I came away feeling a little bit disheartened. I used the term ambivalent on Facebook. I still believe that I might beat the odds, but am realistic enough to understand that they are very formidable, indeed. There may be hard decisions ahead for me, and they will be mine alone to make, but in the meantime, I am beyond happy to have gotten this far along without being sick AT ALL from the disease itself. I mentioned that to the doctor and he agreed that my life outlook has likely played a very big role in making that the case. I intend to maintain the same approach, and certainly hope for the same results. (And, I also plan to continue the Chinese herbal therapy.)

Have you noticed how I have to give you these serious updates from time to time to keep the rhythm and flow of this ongoing saga interesting. Well, that and also to keep you abreast of the whole story. It seems there are more twists and turns to come, and perhaps some bumps and bruises too but, thankfully, we'll get through them together.

Smile with me, for tomorrow is another day that the Lord has made. Let's rejoice and look forward to it with gladness.

<><

Karen

25

May 8, 2013

The Object is to Maintain, Literally at a Cost

Hi folks,

Today was my first day of Avastin maintenance therapy…you know, the medicine that is designed to slow the growth of new blood vessels that would feed the cancer that remains in my lung and liver. Put differently, it should help to hold things at bay and possibly even shrink the tumors further if all goes well over the next several months. The infusion appointment took the better part of an hour and a half, but only because my nurse today was quite the talker. After I got settled in my chair and covered with a comfy blanket, she looked over my computerized records and asked me lots of questions. Our dialogue had a very conversational tone to it, and while I filled her in on many things, since she was one of the nurses I had not yet dealt with in my six chemo treatments, it led to new discoveries on both of our parts.

Among other things, the nurse asked me if anyone had addressed gene markers with me regarding any possible connection between this onset of cancer and my previous experience with both uterine and ovarian cancers way back in 1997. I told her that the subject had not been raised with me by any of the other medical professionals with whom I've dealt these past several months. I can see how it could be useful information for the future, perhaps, but as it relates to this current battle I'm fighting, it doesn't really matter to me. I'm already engaged in it, so I'd rather put my thoughts and energy into the here and now. Since the thought has been planted in my mind though, I will likely address it with my doctor at some point in the future, just out of curiosity.

Once some of those questions were out of the way, and the other patients in her foursome had received whatever attention they also required, we got down to the business of inserting the infusion needle. This nurse was the first one who chose to put it in my hand rather than in my wrist or arm. That made good sense to me considering I have these big, blue, protruding veins all over the backs of my hands that would be better placed on the bulging head of a Pixar super villain. Other nurses had used veins in my wrists or lower arms. Those are not nearly so prominent, so maybe they were just showing their skilled marksmanship with the needles.

Anyway, the nurse popped the needle right on in, taped it up real good, got the saline drip going, and said she'd be back momentarily with the Avastin. She said she had to run to the pharmacy (apparently in one of the nearby rooms of the clinic) to get it. True to her word, she was back within just a couple of minutes. I reviewed my name, birth date and the drug name on the plastic pouch and she plugged it into my little needle and tube contraption. I was a happy little camper and decided to read some articles online on my cell phone to pass the time. You see, I'd forgotten to bring a book, and have opted not to cough up the money for an iPad or even a Kindle so far. You can tell me what you think of those decisions. I can take it. Surely, many of you have strong opinions on the matter.

Once I got underway with my first article, I felt part of my hand beginning to go numb, but I figured it was just because it had a needle stuck in it with strong drugs coursing through my veins. Before too long, however, I moved my hand from where I had placed it atop the blanket covering my lap and saw that a diluted mixture of my blood mixed saline was running all across the back of my hand and spilling out onto the blanket. I calmly said, "Mayday...mayday...I think we have a little problem here." The nurse gave me her undivided attention and grabbed a paper towel for me to hold over my hand while she rapidly donned a pair of latex gloves. She said that one of the small connections among the various tubes was apparently not tight, and she quickly cleaned me up, replaced the soiled blanket with a clean one, and got everything all working properly once more.

I was applauded for noticing the situation quickly so we did not lose much, if any, of the Avastin that was intended to go inside me and not serve as a rinse over the outside of my hand. After all, this stuff costs upwards of $10,000 per bag. Whoa baby! I didn't know that before. So, I've already gotten about $70,000 worth of just that one drug. The nurse said it is only good for up to 8 hours after it is mixed up in the pharmacy, so it wouldn't be such a good thing to mess things up and lose part of a dosage. I told her I would understand if she isn't there the next time I come for a treatment. If I hear anyone mention that she was such a good employee until "the incident," I'll understand completely…of course, I'm only kidding.

Other than that, I'm off to a good start of this new period in my cancer journey. Now, about 5 weeks out from my last chemo treatment, I can tell a very noticeable difference in my hands and feet. Well, really in my whole body with regard to the neuropathy's dissipation. It is by no means gone, but the worst of the itching seems to be leaving and I have begun walking each day now. I can walk at least ½ mile at a time before stopping to rest my feet for a bit. Even then, they are not requiring icing any more, nor are my hands. It is so nice to be returning to more of a state of normalcy again.

Also, I guess I can tell you that what caused me to take a little step back last week when I talked with Dr. Ray about my liver MRI results was his answer to the length of time Avastin therapy would probably hold off renewed cancer growth. I had no preconceived expectation on that answer, but when he came back with 3-4 months…or even 5-6 months, well, I kind of thought that seemed pretty short, indeed. I mean, that barely takes me through the coming summer before the cancer growth might resume. Of course, there are a few good things to remember, and it only took me a day or so to get my mind back to these thoughts. First, my tumors are going down in size, not up, and that is good. I'm continuing to do a two-pronged attack, using both American and Chinese medicine, and I believe that gives me a stronger battle plan. Three, absolutely every individual is different in his or her physiological and psychological makeup and this makes a big difference in the outcome of treatments. Finally, I have an international army of prayer warriors and a God who hears and answers prayer. So, that puts me in a pretty darned good place.

I was just thinking about something a few days ago...something that may surprise many, or perhaps all of you. I actually feel grateful for this experience. It's teaching me a lot, and giving my life a new meaning. It's not always an easy route I'm taking, and I don't always react well to others along the way, but hopefully even those who are sharing the trip with me are gleaning new insights and maybe they'll forgive me if I act irritable every once in a while.

Next time, I really hope to show you a photo or two of my new hair beginning to grace this orb sitting on top of my neck. You know, I just have to go for these strange turns of phrase. By the way, anyone want to place bets on color and texture? I can tell you, I'm pretty eager to find out.

<><

Karen

26

May 16, 2013
A Top Ten Finish

Hi folks,

I decided it was time for a little more pictorial proof that I'm hanging in there and forging ahead with my grand scheme to beat this cancer bully. You know, it's that same one that has punched me in the gut, er perhaps better put in the chest...but also the one that is taking many body blows from me. I'm not going to passively lie down and take a beating the way bullies would wish. No, the way I'm fighting back, in part, is to continue doing all the things I normally do and not letting this interlude throw me off my stride.

In fact, striding is what I'm going to tell you about in this update. You see, each spring, my company holds a 1-mile fun run/walk in order to increase employee attention to fitness and well-being. Last year, the first year I participated and when I was purportedly healthy, I came in third in the walking division. Heck, I didn't even know it was a race until I saw the two who beat me to the finish literally fly off the starting line. Once they took the lead, I held my own to stay with them, but there was simply no way for me to gain on them. They were good, really good! But I'm nothing if not competitive, so I blew the rest of the field away just because I could.

This year, it turned out that I had completed the end of my sixth chemotherapy cycle less than three weeks before the race was held on May 15. The neuropathy that had plagued me throughout the chemo treatments had reached its zenith by the sixth cycle in mid-April. At that point, it was difficult for me to walk more than ¼ mile before my feet would "kick up" so severely with the itching that I could barely race indoors to land them on ice fast enough to calm them from driving me completely insane. Of course, insanity is, to some extent, rather subjective, so you may feel that I was already nearly there anyway and just needed a little nudge to make the trip complete.

Anyway, to my great pleasure, over the past two weeks or so, the itching part of the neuropathy has begun to diminish rapidly, and I had begun increasing my walk lengths with my dog Bella every couple of days. I had gone more than a mile on a couple of occasions by the 15th, so I was pretty sure that I would be able to complete the race reasonably well. Considering what these past few months had done to my body (steroids caused weight gain, severe itching, constant sinus drainage, inability to maintain normal exercise routine due to neuropathy, etc.), I knew that I could not likely expect to reach the top three as I had last year. I did, however, think it might be realistic to aim for the top ten. So, this became my single-minded goal.

The weather was supposed to be warm and sunny but, instead, it was just a little bit cool and overcast with even a few raindrops trying to dampen the road before us (all to no avail, fortunately). I had gone out to enter the race with three of my department friends, though they had chosen to take a more leisurely pace themselves once things got underway. So, leaving them aside, I found my way to the front of the pack as we gathered at the starting line. When the signal was given, I had hoped to hold my own with the leaders for as long as possible. That lasted about 14 nanoseconds. I watched 4 people fly at warp speed out in front of me and realized immediately that I could not keep their pace, so I simply put my head down and told myself to relax my breathing and try not to tense my legs too much as I hurriedly marched on.

About 1/3 of the way along, I heard people closing in behind me and before I knew it, three of them passed me. As I watched them move on ahead, I marveled at the fact that they didn't appear to be walking inordinately fast. In fact, one of them, a gentleman, stopped twice to retie one of his shoes, and I still couldn't quite catch him. What the…? Ah well, I was still in eighth place. We had gone out of our parking lot, around a couple of streets and up a little hill to pass an elementary school. Then, a man doing his version of semaphore directed us down the street beyond the school that took us by some Little League baseball fields, through some thick grass to slow our pace further, through a cut in the woods, and back across a different part of our parking lot to the finish line.

I furtively looked over my shoulder a few times, knowing that only three more people passing me would erase my goal of reaching the top ten. I could not let that happen. I saw a man maybe 15 yards behind me. Oh no! I thought about tripping him. I thought about yelling "fire" and sending him off into the underbrush to check it out. I thought about changing my walk into a concerted jog. But those things would be wrong. So, I clenched my teeth, puffed out my chest and shouted silently, "no one is moving me out of 8th place, period!"

I got through the woods, hit the parking lot pavement, race walked up around the building and saw the cheering throngs welcoming me home. The company photographer was in the distance aiming his camera directly at me which,

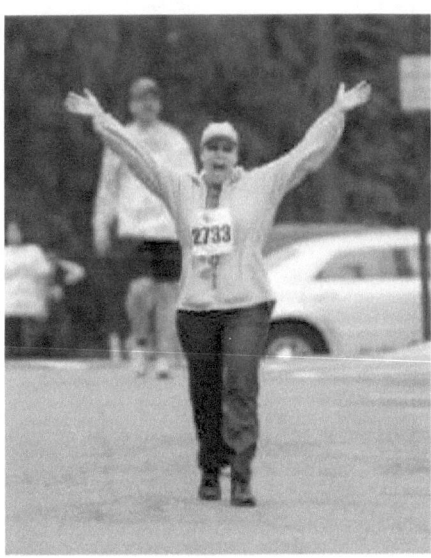

of course, caused me to raise my arms and wave frantically. Then, in the final 20-30 yards, I simply could not help myself. I grabbed my cap, yanked it off and let the sun, which was now out, shine down on me, for I had accomplished my goal in the company Fun Run/ Walk on May 15, 2013. And it was exciting!

It may seem like just a silly little story, but I am truly not kidding when I tell you that I am not going to let this disease hold me down. It helps me to prove over and over to myself that I am the same me with cancer as I was without cancer. Some of you may think that's kind of too bad (she said with a wink), but it's a fact.

<><

Karen

P.S. One quick end-note…I don't have enough hair yet to bother with as I had hoped when I wrote the last update. I am "feeling" more peach fuzz, if not yet "seeing" much. So, my fingers are crossed for enough to show by the start of June. I'll keep you posted.

27

May 23, 2013
Connecting Dots and Wondering

Hi folks,

I woke up early this morning, earlier than I wanted to and earlier than the time my alarm clock told me was wake-up time. Why? Because my body was crying out, "I don't feel so good." The first thing I noticed upon waking was the slight discomfort at the base of my sternum, a twinge, if you will. To most of you, a similar feeling probably wouldn't evoke much reaction, but to me, my mind immediately connected some dots. Let me explain.

For a couple of years before I finally had the correct tests done which brought forth the lung cancer diagnosis, I'd been having recurrent bouts of severe discomfort at the base of my sternum. It was a tight band sensation around my chest which had a particular point, always the same, where I simply felt extreme discomfort, even causing me to run over to immediate care to make sure I was not having a heart attack. It was not a stabbing pain or a burning pain, it was just a tightness and discomfort, and it recurred time and time again. I saw a number of different doctors before finally finding one who, in her attempts to find a gastrointestinal reason for the upset, instead helped me find the cancer I am now fighting.

To my pleasant surprise really, I have not experienced this problem once since the diagnosis clear back at the end of November 2012. This morning, however, I felt just a little bit of the same sensation for the first time in six months. This naturally made me wonder what's going on. As I laid in bed, I thought about two other things I've been experiencing more, or at least noticing more, in the past few weeks. First, the raspy voice that had troubled me for at least the first three months of the period since my diagnosis seems to be returning. It is not nearly as bad or as constant for now as it was then, but it is returning with greater frequency and is certainly quite noticeable. Second, I find it hard to manage a good chest cough when I feel the need to do so. I've never experienced that before, so I don't really know a good way to describe it other than to say it is sort of like a dry cough when a wet cough would feel better. Does that make sense?

While these things were meandering through my mind, my intestines were getting very temperamental. So, I didn't linger on the symptomatic thoughts too much because I had more urgent matters to deal with. I can tell you, however, that even while I battle my disease, and do what I can to lead a normal life, the realities it brings with it are always in the back of my mind. When I might previously have just thought I didn't feel so good for a time, now I sometimes think things like "Is this the beginning of the big slide downward?" or "Wow, is it possible the good 'maintenance' period is already coming to an end?"

Some of you are sure to tell me to simply not allow myself to think these things, but I assure you, it is perfectly normal and human to do so. Put yourself in my shoes, if you can, and I suspect you might have similar thoughts or questions from time to time. They don't stop me from doing fun things like going to ballgames (Well, that's not so fun lately if you're a Nats fan, is it?), riding on a friend's motorcycle up to Gettysburg or continuing to go to work day in and day out. It doesn't stop me from planning some big trips for next fall and late winter (more about that in an upcoming update). It doesn't stop me from walking Bella now that I can walk unimpeded by the itching once again. In fact, I rejoice that I can do all of these things. But, I still know that while I hope to beat this disease, the fact is ever present that I may not…and I do think about it, not with fear, but with wonder.

Recently, I was thinking about these updates I've been sending you all for several months now and how they seem to have somewhat of a roller coaster pattern regarding my use of humor and a bit more seriousness from one to the next. This really is pretty much in keeping with the way my mind is working through this experience. And besides that, I think any story needs its ups and downs, chuckles and challenges, to keep it interesting. Well, if nothing else, I can tell you that from my angle on the inside looking out, it is indeed interesting, to say the least.

Please drop me a line if you feel so inclined. Your notes and messages really do encourage me a great deal.
<><
Karen

28

June 2, 2013
BP Meds, Car Shopping
and Open-Air Topping

Hi folks,

I had my second Avastin maintenance appointment this past Wednesday afternoon. The most memorable part of it was that my nurse, who was also the same one who gave me my first chemo treatment, offered me two Danishes, some fried rice and a nice tasting of grape tomatoes and cucumbers in an oil-based dressing. I guess I should schedule my appointments nearer lunchtime more often, huh?

In my preliminary appointment that day with the nurse practitioner, we found that my blood pressure was rather high again, as it has been nearly every time I've gone to appointments since I began the chemo treatments. The Avastin is the culprit that causes that. This time, it came in at 160/100. That was high enough to warrant my first blood pressure drug ever, a low dose (5 Mg) of Norvasc once a day. I am to read my blood pressure about six hours after taking it each day and keep a chart. Over the first several days since I began the medication, my readings have come in at 161/93, 161/99 and 148/93, 159/94 and 151/94 respectively. I'd like to see it begin to come down a bit more with consistency before too long. If it does not, I'll probably contact my nurse navigator just to keep the doctor apprised in case they want to vary the dosage before my next Avastin appointment on June 19. High blood pressure frequently does not have any noticeable outward symptoms, but it can bring on some serious consequences if not controlled, not least of which is stroke.

Other than this little turn of events, the nurse practitioner told me she didn't feel the changing voice or recurrence of the mild chest tightness/attack were cause for concern regarding tumor growth. I will see her again in three weeks, and then I'll see Dr. Ray the visit after that, five and one half weeks from now. At that visit, I will likely be told when I should schedule the next scan. Until then, I'm going with the assumption that summer is almost upon us and I'm good to go for the warmth, sunshine and playtime that comes with it. As you'll see below, I have added a little excitement to my life this weekend.

I had an unexpected turn of events yesterday morning when I took my 8-year-old car in for its annual state inspection which, this time, also included a required emissions inspection. To my displeasure, it failed both of them. That means that I must either have all the necessary repairs performed and a passing re-inspection completed prior to the end of June in order to renew my tags and registration for the coming year, or I can just say, "not gonna worry about it…gonna go out and get a new car."

I had not been in the car market until about lunchtime yesterday, but now I have made a firm decision to lease a new car in the very near future. This is because last year alone, in only two appointments, I spent close to $2600 in maintenance fees on my older car. That did not include a set of 4 new tires, a couple of oil changes, and the standard stuff. I decided that it simply makes more sense to put all of that maintenance money into a new, healthy automobile rather than pouring more money into an old car at this stage.

You may be wondering why I've chosen to include this brief foray into car-shopping into my "medical" update. The reason is this. I had to decide whether it makes more sense for me to buy or lease a new car right now. I've never leased before, but realize the timeframes are shorter than most people choose when financing purchases, and also the monthly costs are less along the way, although there is no equity built-up in the car at the end of the agreement. The lower the mileage amount written into the contract, the lower the monthly cost. Since my commute to work is literally less than ½ mile each way, I can easily work with a low mileage agreement. Here is where the medical part of the equation comes to play. You know by now that in a much greater sense than is the case for most of us, my long-term future (meaning multiple years vs. multiple decades) is not guaranteed. For that reason, I think a shorter term contract that can still offer me lower monthly payments makes good sense.

I inquired with the first two dealerships I visited about whether there would potentially be a penalty applied if the terms of the lease agreement had to be broken at an early date by my estate. While I don't anticipate this happening, these are the types of practical questions I think about these days. Fortunately, both said that in such a case, the car would simply need to be returned to the dealership and the agreement would come to an end without penalty.

I suspect many of you will be disappointed with me if I don't tell you the cars I have been considering and test driving. Having driven a small SUV for the past 8 years, I've decided to return to the mid-sized sedan market. As a result, I've looked at a Ford Fusion, a Toyota Camry, a Subaru Legacy, a Honda Accord and a Nissan Altima. I've now narrowed things down to two finalists, the Honda Accord and the Toyota Camry. Both have benefits and drawbacks vs. the other, so I haven't made the final determination. It will come soon, however.

Here's something else I did for the first time this past Friday evening since I last did it in early January. I walked Bella outdoors for the better part of a mile without a head covering of any kind. It wasn't entirely intentional. It just so happened that I planned to take her out for a nice walk and had been hatless inside. I leashed her and grabbed the supplies I needed and we made our way outdoors. I was part way down the sidewalk when I realized that I had no hat, scarf or wig on. It felt great! The sun had already set and the weather was nice and warm. My fuzz is getting longer each day, perhaps by the millimeter, but still longer. By next weekend, I'm certain I'll be going topless…that is…no covering on top of my head. Sorry if I caused you the fright of your life there for a second. I know I've been teasing that one along for a few weeks now, but the hair's just been slower coming in than I had expected. This time, it's for real though. Woohoo!

Finally, when I tell you I enjoy receiving your replies in connection to these updates I send out, you might not realize that I don't only receive notes telling me that people are praying for me or find some of the things I write inspiring, though those are lovely thoughts that are passed on to me. Sometimes, I am happy to report, that you send me your prayer requests too. I love to be able to pray for you, just as you do for me. It means we are caring for one another, just as God intends for us to do. This basic message was a part of my pastor's sermon this morning, which was based on part of the Sermon on the Mount. If you ever find yourself feeling down physically or emotionally, try praying for others to improve their outlook on life and yours. What a great way to live!

So, there you have it...a sort of mishmash of thoughts, but stuff that happens in my life as I continue living with and fighting off lung cancer. Pretty normal stuff, eh?

<><

Karen

29

June 10, 2013
Celebrating My New Car,
Hatless and Scarfless

Hi folks,

Today was the first morning in five complete months when I went to work hatless, scarfless and wigless. I

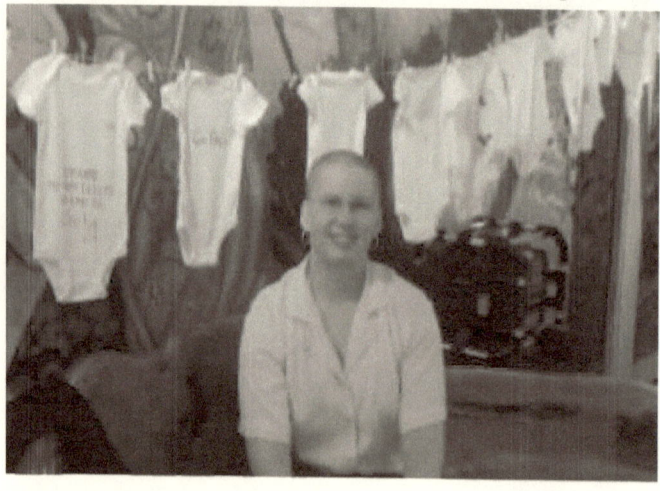

hasten to add, but not hairless. I had begun my new era of openness, to the air that is, this past Saturday, June 8, 2013, when I went to Philadelphia for my nephew and his wife's baby shower.

No one seemed to bat an eyeball at my "spare" look. I hadn't tried to do things up or anything, so when I got ready for work this morning, you might be surprised to know that I had all kinds of trouble getting the part in my hair to hold. Fortunately, no one said much about that. It would have made me more self-conscious, you know? I've posted a few pictures so you'll understand what I'm talking about.

I can tell you that, as we head into summer, it is much more comfortable to go without toppings because they do tend to hold the heat in. I'll just need to be more aware about covering my head when I am out in the sun for any extended period of time. The Washington Nationals are bound to get lots of free publicity from me this season as I wear their caps with pride. Wonder if I could charge an advertising fee?

They even get free publicity on the back of my car with the big curly W magnet I place there so all will know where my baseball loyalties lie. Now, I'll be moving the W from a black car to a shiny, new, white 2013 Honda Accord that I just picked up this evening. My oh my! What a tough decision it was between selecting it or a 2013 Toyota Camry. Everything I read, everyone I talked to and polled, and even my own interests in different features available on each car led me to a completely split decision. The scales were weighing in at 50/50 and by the very smallest of margins, the Accord finally won out. It appeared that nothing was going to tip the balance in a big way, so I had to just bite the bullet and let the side-view camera on the Honda sway me enough to get the darned deal over with.

Now, I am the proud lessee of a beautiful new car, and I will donate a car that has done well by me for eight years to a worthy charity. It's nice to know I can be of help to someone in that way now that I've made the decision that was right for me. You can all enjoy this new car with me as you gaze upon the photo here. Notice my new eyebrows are back.

It appears as though I just came straight from the men's military barber at basic training. Hats off to all of those fine gentlemen who are my comrades in buzzcuts through the years. As for the military ladies, well, I know you're with me in spirit, even if your cuts never quite matched mine.

Some of my foreign friends, particularly some of my Compassion International children and also the Moriah ministry in Ethiopia that I have worked with in recent

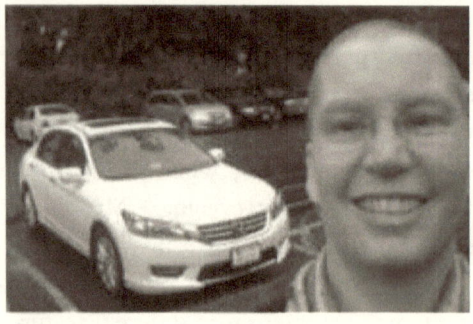

years, have inquired of me in the past few days about my hair loss. Several have not yet seen the photos of me minus my hair, so I will share these new ones with them. And they, along with you all, can jump into the guessing game with me as to how it will eventually turn out. Will it be brown, blonde, auburn…gray? Curly, straight, wavy? What's your best guess? I hope this poll will be more definitive than my car polls were!

As for my actual health during this past week, there is little of note to report. It seems I've had more frequent intestinal upsets in the mornings over the past month or so than I'd had all the way through chemotherapy, but usually some over the counter meds and giving myself an hour or so to get through the problems seems to adequately take care of things. Also, my blood pressure seems to have come down a very small amount, though not much. That's better than staying at the same elevated heights or rising still further, right? I'm charting the progress and will address that when I go in for my third Avastin appointment next week. Seeya next time.

<><

Karen

30

June 19, 2013
Another Avastin Appointment

Hi folks,

I'm back and opening with a representative photo from all of those chemo infusion days that have morphed into Avastin-only treatment days that happen every three weeks. The difference from then until now is that, as you will surely note, I am actually awake during the current treatments. The rest…well, it's the same. I make myself comfortable in the recliner with a pillow and blanket, and just let the little tube with the expensive liquids flowing through it into my veins do its thing.

Today, I had a new infusion nurse whom I had not met before. That may give you an idea of how big this infusion center is, for I've had different nurses all but twice, I think, over the nine different treatments I've received so far. She was pleasant and highly skilled, as they all are. She even chuckled when I suggested that I would prefer the liquid gold pouring into my veins be poured into my wallet instead. She may just have been humoring me, of course. I like that.

Prior to the actual infusion, I always get labs done… that is, blood tests and a urinalysis to test for all kinds of things, making sure each element tested falls within proper ranges. Occasionally, one of the many results will fall slightly outside of the range, but unless it is a significant finding, the doctor and nurses don't seem to get concerned, so I don't either.

Following the labs, I meet with the nurse practitioner, physician assistant, or the doctor. Today, once again, I met with the nurse practitioner. I showed her the blood pressure and pulse readings I'd been charting for the past three weeks since I began taking Nor-vasc. My BP is still

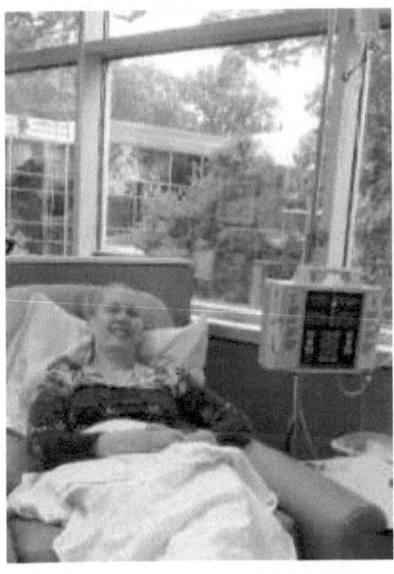

generally reading higher than was the case prior to this whole period of cancer treatments, but the Norvasc has seemed to bring it down slightly on a consistent basis, e-nough that we did not feel the need to increase the dosage for now. I will continue to chart the readings each day, just to keep an eye on things.

Yesterday, when I picked up my bi-weekly supply of herbal supplements (that awful tasting tea drink and the American ginseng capsules) from Dr. H, I asked her to tell me how I am to know if her treatments are actually helping me. She said that cancer is not static. It will either grow or retreat. If the next scan shows it regressing, she may reduce the amounts of the herbal supplements I am now taking. So, in correlation to that notion, I asked the nurse practitioner how long I will likely continue with Avastin therapy if we find that the tumors continue to shrink in upcoming scans. Avastin is not given as an agent to shrink tumors, but instead it is intended to keep them from progressing for as long as possible. Anyway, the answer to my question was unavoidably nebulous. She did, however, say it could go on for quite some time but would eventually need to be stopped, like any of the cancer drugs, because there comes a time when they can begin to cause harm simply due to long-term use. I think this, in part, is one of the reasons for the lab tests that are run before each and every treatment.

After I included a photo in the last update showing my hair and eyebrows are beginning to return, I failed to mention that my eyelashes are back too. Well, the eyelashes are still short, but they are indeed there again. And, the eyebrows are rather light, but they, too, are there. In fact, I never realized this before, but I think they have some wave or curl in them, thus making them rather unruly. I believe I may need a little dab of Brylcreem to settle 'em down. Or maybe some Dippity-Do. Well, maybe not.

Anyway, you'll really understand now that I am truly trying to share the good, the bad and the ugly with you through these updates when you see the photo of my eyes included here. I wanted you to notice the brows and lashes of which I speak, but I would very much appreciate

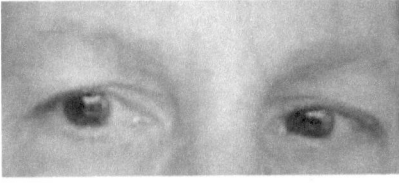

if you could avert your gaze from the wrinkles. They are surely not mine, but some inexpert pho-

tographer's notion of a practical joke.

Oh, and by the way, I must say I was rather surprised at the number of people guessing my impending hair color to be gray. I guess they'd seen the eye close up before I had. Still, I strongly suspect they will be wrong, though it still seems far from certain what the end result will be. So far, it does not look as though it will have those same auburn overtones as before, though I hope I'm wrong on that. If the "grays" turn out to be right, I may do a future update from the hair color makeover salon. Don't make me go there...PLEASE. Otherwise, I might have to finally start acting my age, and that would be a real tragedy, don't you think?

<><

Karen

31

June 29, 2013
Goodbye Tucker Tucson
and Leveling with the Doc

Hi folks,

Parting is such sweet sorrow... Okay, so I plagiarized that little phrase from someone just a bit more famous than me, but it embodies such meaning. You see, yesterday morning, about 7 a.m., I said goodbye to a friend of eight years. I had come to know him as Tucker Tucson only days before, for I had been under the illusion that her gentleness and comforting nature, not to mention a lovely sound system, meant that indeed she was a girl. Turns out I was wrong. Cars, it seems, do not have gender specific features that would make this more obvious, so Tucker took no offense at my lapse in judgment. After all, we were friends, pals, and confidantes.

This is why, though I sent him off to an eventual new home with a U.S. military veteran who needs him and will care for him, I got just a tad misty in the morning. I saw the tow truck pull up. I handed over the keys saying, "He runs fine, so you can drive him right out of his parking space to load." Then, I raced inside to get his Title and the second set of keys. By the time I returned, he sat, like a proud warrior, atop the flatbed truck. My emotions were swirling, so much so that I never even thought to get a final photograph. I just signed him over, gazed with melancholy eyes, and said "Bye Tucker. I'll miss you."

With that, he was gone. I know, I know. Tucker Tucson was only a car, but he had served me well. And I will have happy memories of this little SUV who hauled Bella and me about, who could park in the tiniest of spaces, and who could do donuts inside of donuts because his turn ratio was so tight. And now, he will continue his service to another fortunate soul.

Okay, so the car story has nothing to do with providing a medical update on my cancer situation, does it? Well, let's move on then, shall we? For the past week plus, I've been experiencing what seems like near constant tiredness. Why is that? Does it relate to my disease? I am choosing to believe that there is probably no connection, but that I simply need to change my habits, behave myself if you will, and go to bed at a decent hour. I guess some of us need more than 5-6 hours of sleep per night, whether we are willing to do what it takes to get it or not.

With this new insight in mind, I decided that I would not only sleep in today (it's Saturday, so I could legitimately do so), but I snuggled back into bed late in the afternoon for a pleasant and needed nap. My colleagues at work will surely nod knowingly when I tell you that it is nearly a daily ritual for me to come back from lunch and gently grab their attention only to say with complete sincerity, "I need a nap!" I even have in mind where I could stash a nice sleeping mat in relative darkness (right underneath my desk and back by the wall). You can see that I've put some real thought into this, but I suspect those paying me to work might have other notions, so I have refrained from taking it to the next step…so far.

When I visit the cancer specialists on July 10 for my next Avastin appointment, however, I will raise this point with the nurse practitioner when she asks me how things are going. I will also tell her about something that has been troubling my left hand for a couple of months now. I have been experiencing pain in the knuckle on my little finger and the big joint at the base of my thumb. In fact, at times, depending on what activity I am using my hand to accomplish, I have even wondered if I might have broken my little finger, or if I might yet do so if I continue to use it to perform said activity. The pain and discomfort doesn't go away in either finger and I suspect it is arthritis. There is not much outward sign of change to these fingers, though perhaps there is a slight amount of swelling in the little finger joint.

These two things are not likely connected to the lung cancer that remains lurking inside me, but that is only my guess and assumption. Better to let my doctor and his associates know so they can have a more complete sense of what is going on with me physically, right? They might know something I don't. Well, that's the idea, right? Doctors are supposed to know things we lay people don't when it comes to health and wellness and treatment of pain and disease.

With that thought in mind, I've decided, with the wise counsel of a good friend that I must get past my uneasiness about telling Dr. Ray and his team about the herbal treatments I have been taking since February 19th of this year. When I asked about adding a complementary treatment of this sort to the chemotherapy they had me on, they advised against it. You probably recall my mentioning this some time ago. Anyway, as a result, I chose to overrule their advice and go forward with the treatments, directed by Dr. H, an OMD (Oriental Medicine Doctor) and registered herbalist. For some reason, I had what is probably an unwarranted fear that my doctor might tell me he could not continue my treatment if I would not listen to his instruction on this matter, and I did not want to have this projected confrontation. So, I simply went about doing both therapies.

I continue to think I am doing the right thing by doing complementary therapies. In fact, I believe that for at least the first few months that I did the herbal treatments, they played a significant role in changing and maintaining my positive outlook on the potential outcome of my cancer journey. While those beliefs have settled some now and I am feeling less certain, I am not yet ready to discontinue the herbal treatments. This is a fairly big deal for me because they are not covered by my medical insurance and the cost is not cheap. I look forward to learning when my next PET scan will be, because if it shows continued shrinkage of the tumors, I will believe the herbs are likely a large part of the cause. This is because, as I have previously noted, the Avastin is not designed to shrink the tumors, but mainly to keep them from being metabolically active.

See, I knew if I worked at it, I could give you a real medical update, and so, in the end, I did.

<><
Karen

32

July 13, 2013
Rocking Out with Sir Paul and Other Things

Hi folks,

I held off writing this update because I knew what loomed ahead for me on the evening of July 12, 2013. Even though I grew up in the era that brought about rock 'n roll's larger than life legends, I was never a particular fan of the genre. There was one performer, however, a classic rock 'n roller, who I included in my personal category of musical favorites. And I got to go and see him perform live last night at Nationals Stadium. Yes, Sir Paul McCartney was in town with his Out There tour. He played and sang for two hours and 42 minutes…non-stop. This man is 71 years old, or young if you'd prefer, and even at that age, he bounced, strummed, plinked, sang and simply applied his charm to the sold-out audience there to cheer him on. I marveled at how he could still muster the huge amount of energy it takes to perform a concert like that on an extended tour that on this night included 36 of his best known hits from the 1960s all the way through to the present. He offered special memories of and songs dedicated to Jimi Hendrix, John Lennon, George Harrison and his former wife Linda Eastman.

Toward the end of the concert, the band started into "Live and Let Die." As most of you will know, when the power comes in after the first title phrase, it was the perfect time for pyrotechnical explosions. Yes, the fire cannons went off on stage, and fireworks shot into the air above the stadium. Anyone who may have been lulled down memory lane prior to that was catapulted into heart pounding euphoria. I must tell you, however, that there was one little drawback late in the evening. It was actually somewhat humorous, though still frustrating. During the first of his encore numbers, Paul returned to the stage with an acoustic guitar to render a truly beautiful rendition of "Yesterday"…all the while a lady sitting directly behind me was singing along at the top of her lungs and not even remotely close in pitch or tonality. I was glad that she was so enjoying herself, but a little sad that she was ruining this beautiful ballad for all those sitting near her.

I guess that's enough about the concert, but if you get the chance to take in one of McCartney's tour dates, by all means, do it. It'll lift your spirits and make you smile.

Now, on to more mundane things. Ha! You knew that had to come, didn't you? I have begun playing my trombone a little bit once again, at least enough to regain some degree of competence in preparation for a couple of church dates where I've been invited to play. A week from tomorrow, on July 21, I'll be joining the congregants at Bethany United Methodist Church in central Pennsylvania and providing some special music during their morning service. This is the same church my grandfather, a 25-year pastor there in the middle of the last century, helped to build. It pleases me that they wanted me to come and share whatever talent I have in their morning worship. Later in the summer, or perhaps in the fall, I'll play at my own church here in metropolitan Washington, DC.

One thing that surprised me, even though perhaps it should not have, as I began practicing again recently, was that I have very little "wind" to hold out long notes. Well, not just long notes, but even moderately long notes. Well, not just moderately long notes, but even medium length notes. This is not so good, and my first inclination was to blame it on my disease. But as I've thought more about it, I suspect it has much less to do with that, and much more to do with the fact that I am so out of shape from not having exercised the muscles needed to play the trombone with any skill. Like any athlete or actor or singer, I simply need to put in the preliminary work that is required to excel at my craft.

You see what happened to me, even though I may often give the pretense of not letting cancer dominate my thoughts? In reality, it is ever present in the forefront of things in my life. That doesn't mean I dwell on it, but whenever my brain must contemplate a way to do something, or reasons why something is occurring, the grid of possibilities that immediately forms always includes cancer in one panel. Then, I either gravitate toward it or away from it as I ponder the outcome of my dilemma. Interesting, huh?

This past Wednesday, I had another Avastin

treatment. In my visit with the nurse practitioner prior to the infusion, I informed her of my frequent tiredness over recent weeks and inquired as to whether this might be caused by the heightened blood pressure due to the Avastin. She said that was not at all likely. So, I made the obvious and almost certainly correct deduction. I need to improve my sleep habits and go to bed earlier. Doesn't that sound easy? Well, doesn't it? I keep telling myself that as I seemingly do just the opposite. Maybe I need some encouragement on this front, for nighttime is my time. I like nighttime. I don't like early morning nearly so well. What to do? What to do?

The other thing that happened as I conversed with the nurse practitioner was a relief. It was almost laugh-out-loud funny to me. I had decided that whichever practitioner I met with, the doctor, nurse practitioner, physician assistant, whomever, I was going to come clean on the herbal supplements I've been taking for five months now. And so I did. Near the end of our brief appointment, I simply said, "Oh, and by the way, though they aren't really drugs, I have been taking herbal supplements for some time now." I handed her the list Dr. H had given me of herbs that are in the tea I drink each morning and night. She quickly scanned over it and said "okay, that's fine." Maybe this should be instructive to all of us, for I had projected my assumed reactions onto the medical staff for months, which is why I resisted telling them about the herbs.

Dr. H had informed me that most western doctors are not very receptive to herbal treatments, and both Dr. Ray and his assistants had explicitly recommended against this type of complementary therapy. So, I thought I'd be body slammed if I admitted to going over and above their advice. In the end, the opposite happened. Apparently, they look for St. John's Wort and a few specific herbs which create red flags, none of which were on my list, so I was, in effect, good to go. That took a load off of my mind, for it had been uncomfortable to constantly know I was concealing something from my medical team, even though I felt entirely confident with what I was doing.

Now you know one of the little secrets I'd been withholding. Well...you knew it right along huh? Now it's your turn. Pour out your heart. Send me your secrets. I won't share them any farther than this massive and growing readership. I promise.

<><

Karen

33

July 22, 2013

Celebrating My Birthday and Planning Trips

Hi folks,

One more year under my belt…which is why I don't wear swimming suits in public these days. It brings terror to the hearts of children, at least those who aren't heard clapping and shouting, "Mommy, look. There's Shamu!" Ah well, I can always downsize to Flipper. After all, she was a pretty smart and sweet ol' gal in her day. Now, I'm looking to achieve somewhere in the vicinity of 30 more birthdays before all is said and done. Oh, and until today I shared my birthday with the likes of that most famous of all men. Who is Alex Trebek? Former Senate Majority Leader Bob Dole was also a July 22nd baby. Now, the future king of England and my great niece will also share this rather terrific day. I believe they chose their arrival date well.

Yesterday, I made my first appearance with instrument in hand at the front of a church in well over a year. As I mentioned in the last update, I was invited to bring my own little musical touch to three hymns being sung in a service dedicated to two 20th century hymn writers, Natalie Sleeth and Shirley Erana Murray. I found that, after a bit of practice over the last couple of weeks, my form did improve in terms of regaining some degree of stamina as well as better tone quality. Go figure…practice brings progress. Who knew? People even complimented me and told me they liked what they heard. I chose to believe them, then smiled and thanked them in return for the opportunity to play in morning worship at Bethany United Methodist Church, Marysville, PA, on July 21, 2013.

You know what one of the best things is now that I

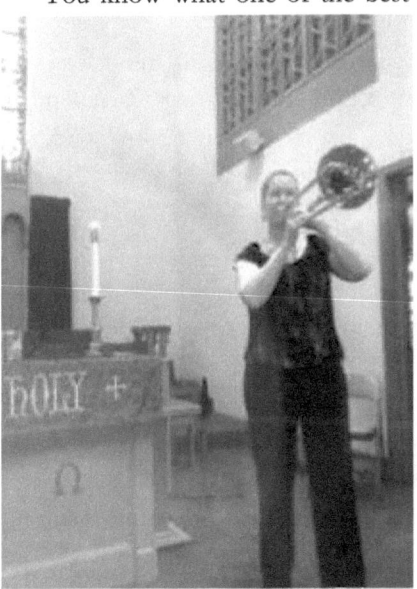

am well past the end of the rounds of chemo from a few months ago? Even with very short hair that is still in the early stages of growing back, I think I can safely say that no one, NO ONE, thinks I'm sick. Even those who know the disease I'm battling do not see me as sick, and those who don't know would never guess. I love that! I look healthy, act healthy, and think healthy. Maybe we'll find out with my next scan, which I hope will happen in August, that indeed I AM HEALTHY in a complete sense. Time will tell.

Meanwhile, I got final word last week that I will be able to participate in Compassion International's November sponsor tour to Haiti. Many of you know that I've been sponsoring Compassion children for 14 years now and, in fact, my Haitian boy has been with me for the full 14 years. He is now in his final year in the Compassion program. I visited him in 2003 when he was a very shy 9-year-old. Now, he has grown into a handsome young man of 19. I promised him when I was spending that wonderful visit with him, taking him into a pool and the ocean for the first time in his life, that I would try very hard to return before he graduated, and this is my opportunity to do just that.

This trip and others have been on my mind for some time now, and I have been contemplating when I might need to carry them out based on my health condition. After a brief consultation with my doctor way back in April, we decided that Haiti in November looked like a good bet. The tumors were metabolically silent, or nearly so, and my outlook appears bright for now. The next two trips I'm already beginning to plan are a little less certain, only because it's hard for any of us to know what our future will hold many months out. Of course, this is a little bit more of the case for me. Still, if international adventure is one of the things that fires up one's heart and mind, as it does for me, then I think preparing to fill my passport with stamps from abroad is a part of my healing regimen.

With that in mind, I will only say that my plans are coalescing for a 3-week trip down under to New Zealand and Australia in February of 2014. They will become my 23rd and 24th countries visited. And I'm hoping very much to return to Ethiopia early next summer to attend the university graduations of two of my Compassion children there. Imagine that. These two young adults who grew up in a climate of poverty unknown to most Americans have worked hard to take advantage of the opportunity they've been given. They are setting and achieving educational goals, and preparing for a better future – one in which they will glorify God as they provide for their families and seek to improve their communities and even their entire nation.

So, you can see, my life is full…and in its own way, I even count my cancer as a blessing. It allows me to communicate with so many people who only a year ago were probably not even on my radar. I have had the chance to educate others through these writings in ways I never would have guessed, ways that make us think, or laugh, or feel a degree of frustration, or even itch (!). I believe this is all for good. And I remain always thankful to God for every blessing. Amen.

<><
Karen

34

August 4, 2013

Odds and Ends

Hi folks,

I'm going to do something entirely out of the norm for me. Something that may cause you to jump for joy and shout hallelujah. You may even break out the party hats and fire up the leftover July 4th combustibles. Surely, you will be happier than you've been in…well…moments.

This update is going to be nothing more than a bullet list, and a short one at that. Why, you may ask. Look at bullet number five for the definitive answer.

And away we go.

1. Due to my consistently high blood pressure over the past six weeks, even though we've been treating with a low dose (5 mg) of Norvasc, Dr. Ray decided it would be best to double the dosage. If that does not bring it more in line with where we want it, we'll try a different medication. So far, the higher dosage does seem to be making inroads.

2. My next scan, which will be a chest/abdomen/pelvis CT with contrast, is scheduled for August 15 at 10 a.m. EDT. I will get the results when I visit with Dr. Ray on August 21 in the early afternoon just prior to my next Avastin appointment. As usual, I am very eager to get this test done, not because I expect anything in particular to result, but because it is the only way I have to know where things currently stand inside my body with regard to this ol' cancer.

3. Over the past month, since my hair has begun to come in thick and medium brown with even a hint of wave on top, I've received many compliments from people, most especially from women. The neat thing is, they have not been compliments about my hair growing back, but simply about the fact that they think it looks good and even stylish in this very short form. It is exceptionally soft and super simple in the care department. So, I am beginning to wonder if I should keep it very short on purpose. I never expected this to even become a consideration. So, I am wavering for the moment.

4. I've decided to get down to serious business about trying to put my cancer journey into book manuscript form and see if I can direct it to a publisher who will agree that it can potentially find a significant audience and serve to encourage many who are fighting cancer or caring about others who are. My infusion nurse this past Wednesday told me another of her patients at my clinic recently had a book published about breast cancer, so...why not me too, right?

5. Finally, the most important bullet for this update. I'm tired. Have been for days...weeks...months. But for the

sake of this short piece, we'll stick with days. We've talked about my needing more sleep. Well, it remains truer than ever, and as I prepared to write another update a few days ago, I told friends on Facebook that my energy had run off with the milkman. It seems, they've now gotten engaged. Every now and again I have dates with new energies, but so far, none have turned into long-term relationships. I'm working on that.

So, I bid you adieu for this time. Looking forward to hearing from you, and in the meantime, wishing you all well in your daily lives.

<><

Karen

35

August 8, 2013
Preparing My Mind and Soul

Hi folks,

I decided to put out another update a little sooner than I often do just because I think I have something to say this evening. You may recall, a couple of months back I talked about the attack in my chest that caused me concern because of its similarity to those recurrent attacks I'd had leading up to my diagnosis. Both the nurse practitioner and my doctor told me they did not feel it was likely cause for concern. This was, at least in part, because it had only happened two or three times over the last couple of months after not having occurred at all while I went through chemo treatments. That has, unfortunately, changed over the past week. It seems that, since I saw Dr. Ray on July 31, I've had these attacks at least 3-4 times, with today's being the most severe of the bunch.

So, even though I said in my last update on August 4 that I have no expectations of what might turn up in this next scan that will be performed a week from today, my mind is focusing a lot more on that now. While no one could know for certain that these attacks a couple of years ago were related to the subsequent finding of lung cancer, none of the tests and treatments tried prior to the final CT scan and biopsy that led to that diagnosis had offered any answers...and the attacks continued. They were always in the same location, always had the exact same symptoms with varying degrees of severity. Now, they are back -- the exact same attacks that make me quite uncomfortable and cause me to simply not feel very good. I am not unable to function. I am not nauseous. I just get a tightness and discomfort in the middle of my chest.

A friend told me it was okay to feel fear, and she gave me many Biblical examples to draw upon. To be honest though, I don't feel fear in mortality matters, though I certainly am mighty curious and eager to find out what is going on inside me. If there is fear, and I really hate that word, it is in simply not looking forward to the prospect of feeling sick more than I feel well, and of possibly not getting to undertake some of the travel I am planning. I am not throwing in the towel...just pondering in print.

Some of you may immediately want to tell me that I am jumping the gun on these thoughts, that surely this is nothing. I hope I may be able to share something here that will help all of us as we deal with family, friends and acquaintances who must deal with difficult situations. Take your cues from, in this case, me. You know, I don't talk about these serious types of thoughts very often, so when I do, allow me to express myself, and know that what I am saying is important. Even my doctor can never know exactly what I feel inside my body and/or my soul. It is an experience that no one else can completely share. I am not looking for sympathy. I am just trying to help you understand in the best way I can.

Part of this cancer journey involves preparing one's mind and soul for whatever lies ahead. I can't shy away from any eventuality because, in the end, I must face wherever the road takes me. I wish this were not part of the journey, but the fact is I think about cancer, my cancer, all the time. There I said it. Did you know that before? Perhaps not, but I think it is surely true for most folks who must deal with a serious ailment like this if we are honest about it.

I think about the things I want to do yet...write my book, write more hymns, travel down under, see my Compassion kids again and simply make a positive difference in this world. But, I also think about what needs to be in my will, how I would like my funeral service to be handled, and what I hope my legacy might be. To some, these may sound like morbid thoughts, but to me, they bring a degree of comfort, and I think are things all of us might be well advised to think about in the quiet of our own minds at some point. It helps us to focus our lives, even when we are not facing perilous medical possibilities.

I wasn't quite sure when I was going to share this hymn I wrote a few years after I'd faced down ovarian and uterine cancers. Now feels like the right time, so I hope you will enjoy it and take the words to heart. It has a melody and I hope to share that with you sometime soon.

He's Always There

I know my Lord. He set me free,
When life's wounds would soon have conquered me.

The words were clear. "You're sick, it's true."
But Jesus said, "I'll make you new."

Chorus

With a tear in my eye, and in His voice,
Christ Jesus said, "I am the choice.
Lay your trust at my feet. Then turn away.
Your work's not done, nor is your play."

Chorus

"Go out to the world, and to those you know.
Plant the seeds of my love, and help them grow,
For even in trial, hurt and despair,
You need not ask, I'm always there."

Chorus

Chorus
I thank you Jesus, great physician.
You spared me for my one true mission.
Use me for your greater glory.
Count me in your wondrous story.

    I hope you find these updates worthwhile. It is
important for me to share them with you, and I remain
ever grateful for your constant encouragement, love and
prayers.
<><
Karen

36

August 21, 2013
Good Results and Reflections on Life

Hi folks,

Good news! The Avastin "Maintenance" Therapy seems to be doing just that...helping maintain the status quo. I decided to wait until today to write another update because it was to be another in the string of results-oriented appointments following my periodic scans. The last one, in late April, showed a small amount of shrinkage in the tumors in my right lung and liver. As noted in the August 8 update, I was getting more and more curious to know if anything untoward might be going on in there because of the restarted chest attacks. The answer, it seems, is that we still don't know the derivation of those doggone attacks in the center of my chest, but at least it may not be connected with the cancer. The size of the small tumors in my lung and liver, while increased a tiny amount, are said to be "not significantly changed."

I visited with the nurse practitioner again today. I asked her whether a person can potentially live with malignant tumors inside their lung and liver for not just years but decades. While she readily assured me that this disease, which is considered incurable, can become "chronic" for extended periods, she wasn't quite comfortable with offering the idea that it could stay that way for multiple decades. In a previous conversation with her, I came to the conclusion that barring something even more precipitous, like an automobile accident, or flesh-eating bacteria, or some other horrible circumstance, this disease is likely to get me in the end…but it could be quite a ways down the road yet. Probably, many of you are thinking that's what you've been believing and assuming right along, and certainly what you have been praying for. I would like to simply say that God is hearing our prayers and blessing me with good health (and also a nice, thick head of soft brown hair), despite the potential for it to be otherwise.

One question I don't dwell on, though I do think about, is why am I doing so well in my battle when others who are equally focused on fighting their own cancer wars, and who have strong and loving support systems, are losing ground. I don't think there is or can be an adequate answer to that other than that every single case has its own infinite variables, and thus no two outcomes can or will ever be the same. As the book of Ecclesiastes says in chapter three, "There is a time for everything, and a season for every activity under the heavens: a time to be born and a time to die…" I believe this completely, and because of this, I can go on from day to day knowing that even if I eventually must deal with the more harsh and painful parts of my disease, God's plan will be fulfilled as it relates to my life.

Last weekend, I had the good fortune to be invited to spend a day with thousands of other women at the Verizon Center in Washington, DC attending the Women of Faith conference. One of the speakers helped me zero in on an answer to an age-old question I've grappled with for my entire adult life. I have always wondered where I fit in...what my niche in life is. Indeed, what is my purpose on this planet? Do any of you ever wonder the same thing? Anyway, this woman told the story of a friend of hers who felt strongly called by God to something, though she couldn't quite put her finger on what that something was. She left her high level professional job to try and follow this call wherever it would lead, and found herself doing nothing more than babysitting for the children of her friends for the next year and a half. In time, she found herself becoming more and more frustrated until one day, like a bolt of lightning, she realized that she was fulfilling God's call by nurturing those little children. In turn, that was feeding the souls of their parents. And the snowball effect was continuing outward from the love and care she was simply pouring into three little children.

My understanding of God's call on my own life has been coalescing over the last many years as I have, through His direct intervention, gained an international family of six children (all now young adults) whom I love like my own. By opening my heart to these kids, I have been blessed beyond measure. And now, as a result of my third go-round with cancer, and the most serious yet, I have found the means to engage with hundreds, if not thousands, of people on an ongoing basis in a way that educates and hopefully nourishes all of us in ways we wouldn't have imagined prior to these past nine months. You know, it doesn't take a high-powered executive office, a big bank account, fame and notoriety. It just takes loving God and being open to His will. I feel so honored to be used in His mission field, which is something I simply call my daily life.

One last thing I probably should add...about that fame and notoriety thing, well, I do have a starring role in an upcoming company video production, so I can only say "lookout Hollywood. Karen's on the move."

<><

Karen

37

EPILOGUE

Between August and November of 2013, I continued chugging along in my happy little maintenance mode, mostly feeling good and even more, feeling confident about what my next scan on December 2nd would show. I was so confident, in fact, that I didn't think much about it. This complacency, if you will, even caused me to falter a bit in my writings to the vast throngs following my progress because it seemed there was little to say on the medical front anymore. I knew that was likely to change eventually but...not here, not now.

I will admit, as I got closer to the scan date in early December, my anticipation grew. A bit of anxiety grew right along with it. I can't say why exactly. Perhaps I just had a feeling. Anyway, I went about my normal routine. You know, work, church, playtime on weekends, a little bit of travel to visit family and to see my Compassion boy in Haiti in mid-November. It had been ten years since our last visit and I count myself very blessed indeed to have had this opportunity once more. Then Thanksgiving came and went. And finally, the day was upon me.

December 2nd arrived and I eagerly walked into the radiology office for the CT scan that would direct my path forward. As always, before I walked out, the desk attendant handed me a CD with all of the pictures on it. When I arrived home, I pushed it into the computer drive and looked intently at the images, wishing I had a single clue how to read them correctly, but knowing it was a pointless exercise. I would simply have to wait the three days until I visited with Dr. Ray and get the results directly from him.

On December 5th, I was escorted into an examining room where I waited for the doctor. Almost as soon as he entered…well, after he politely greeted me…he got right to the point. The tumor on my liver had nearly doubled in size since the last scan in August, and that meant that the Avastin maintenance therapy had completed its run.

While I hated this result, I am glad to have a doctor who doesn't beat around the bushes and try to ease me into things. He treats me like an educated adult who can both understand medical information he shares with me, and one who can accept and deal with news of this nature. After all, I've done my homework and am well aware of the nature of this disease. So, we immediately began discussing the way forward, which for me meant possible clinical trials or a new round of chemotherapy with a different chemo drug, Taxotere (docetaxol) in this case.

As of January 2014, I began chemotherapy round two. The battle wages on. And I am not giving in. The opponent is fierce, and sometimes it does feel like I'm taking one step forward and two steps back, but my armor remains in place. That is, my physical armor and my spiritual armor. This war is far from over. And in the end, I will be victorious, whatever the outcome.